Need a Hand?

A Home Guide to Common Wrist and Hand Problems

Michael B. Wood, MD

NEED A HAND?: A HOME GUIDE TO COMMON WRIST AND HAND PROBLEMS

1405 SW 6th Avenue • Ocala, Florida 34471 • Phone 352-622-1825 • Fax 352-622-1875
Website: www.atlantic-pub.com • Email: sales@atlantic-pub.com
SAN Number: 268-1250

Library of Congress Control Number: 2020011445

Printed in the United States

PROJECT MANAGER: Crystal Edwards
INTERIOR LAYOUT AND JACKET DESIGN: Nicole Sturk

Table of Contents

Introduction/Preface

The intention of this book is to guide decision-making when dealing with problems arising in the hand and wrist, and especially regarding when and how urgently to seek competent medical attention for a variety of common conditions. It is not intended to be a comprehensive information source for all hand and wrist diseases, nor a do-it-yourself treatment guide. It does, however, contain suggestions for what conditions may warrant initial home treatments or at least delayed medical appointments.

It specifically does not discuss acute injuries (for example: falls, lacerations, major injuries, etc.) that should be evaluated promptly and appropriately by qualified medical professionals.

This book is organized into sections that describe the type of symptoms one might encounter when a hand or wrist problem arises.

It attempts to use language and words familiar to a lay, non-medically trained reader, but also includes medical terminology in parentheses in the event that further study is desired through the internet or library sources.

Lumps and Bumps

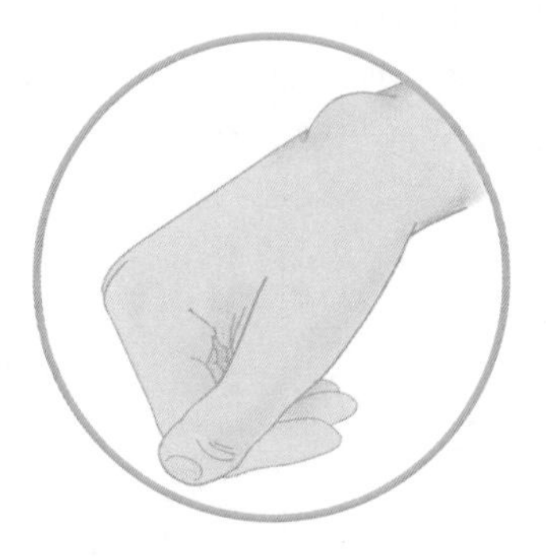

Most lumps and bumps on the fingers, hand, or wrist are due to arthritis, cysts, benign tumors, or infection. Occasionally, they may be a result of a deformity that is birth-related or due to an old bony injury that did not heal in the proper position.

Lumps and bumps due to arthritis are most common. They usually arise gradually and can be painful or tender to the touch. Some of the most frequent locations include:

☞ END JOINT OF THE FINGER (distal interphalangeal joint):

Here, the lumps looks like an enlargement of the entire joint and is referred to as a Heberden's node. It can be painful, but is usually minimally so and the joint is typically somewhat stiff. It is most common in women as they age. Often, a family member has the same condition. The usual concern is that the end joint appears knobby. Although surgical shaving of the enlargement is possible, it is rarely done because it can result in converting a painless condition into one that is painful and may further decrease motion of the joint. Further enlargement of the joint over time usually does not occur. Thus, for most people, simply understanding what this condition is and living with it is the best decision.

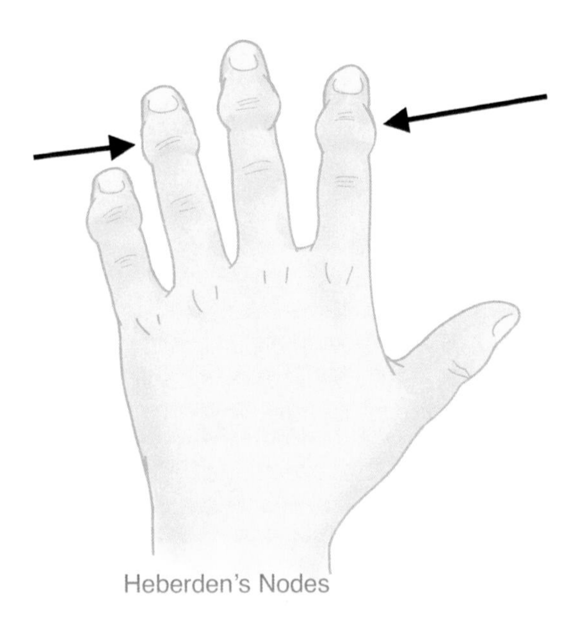

Heberden's Nodes

☞ TOP (dorsum) OF END JOINT OF THE FINGER:

There is a special lump that may look like a water blister very close to the root of the fingernail and is referred to as a mucus cyst. At times, it may cause a groove in the fingernail. It is usually the size of a BB or pea and is hard to the touch. It actually arises from the underlying finger joint. It may be drained with a syringe under sterile conditions, though the cyst often recurs. Therefore, surgery may be necessary to remove it completely. Although it may seem tempting to drain the mucus cyst at home, this should be avoided because of the risk of deep infection in the underlying joint.

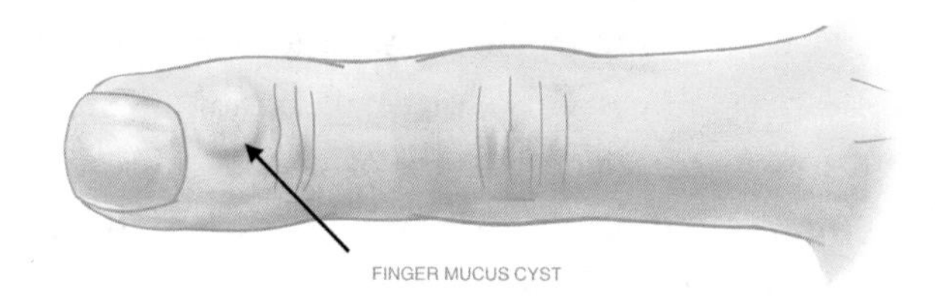

FINGER MUCUS CYST

☞ PALM SIDE OF THE FINGER TIP:

Although not extremely common, a deep hard round bump or nodule may develop some weeks or months after a puncture wound to the fingertip. These are known as epidermoid inclusion cysts and are due to the puncture-injury event driving some surface skin cells into the deeper tissues. Although epidermoid inclusion cysts can occur in any location, they are common around the tip of the finger since this is the most frequent location for a puncture wound from a needle or sharp object. By the time they are recognized, these cysts may have grown to the size of a large pea. They cannot be drained because they are rather solid with a paste-like inner core. Thus, treatment requires surgical removal.

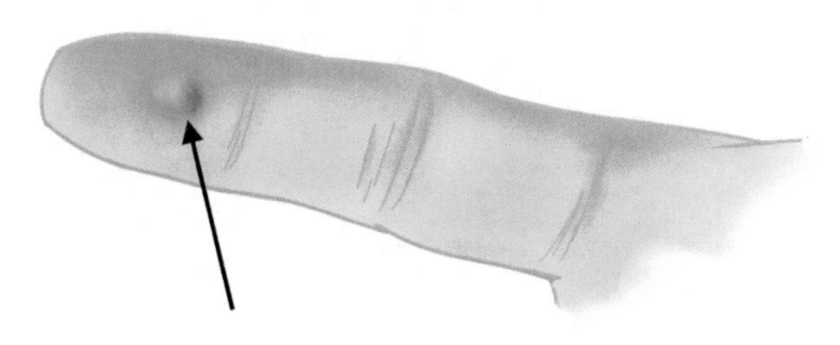

EPIDERMOID CYST OF FINGERTIP

☞ BASE OF THE THUMB:

Arthritic joint changes at the base of the thumb may initially appear as a swollen lump or hard bump. Wear and tear arthritis (osteoarthritis) at the base of the thumb is the most common site for painful arthritis in the hand. Firm pinching or gripping usually makes the pain worse. A frequent complaint is difficulty turning a key in a lock, holding a pen, pushing on stiff buttons, or twisting off jar lids. This condition is most common in women and people over the age of 60. Because arthritis at the base of the thumb is painful and makes gripping and pinching activities difficult, treatment is often necessary to maintain quality of life. The simplest treatment involves the wearing of a brace that supports the wrist and wraps about the base of the thumb (thumb shell splint). This alone may be sufficient treatment for temporary symptoms or for selected aggravating activities, but the use of a brace alone is not a practical solution for extended daytime use. Therefore treatment by a medical professional may be preferable. A doctor may advise an injection of cortisone or other anti-inflammatory agent into the joint or surgery. If surgery is advised, there are several different choices ranging from simple removal of the arthritic wrist bone (trapezium) at the base of the thumb, to an artificial joint implant. The most common surgical procedure is removal of the trapezium and the wrapping of a tendon from the wrist around the base of the thumb (first metacarpal).

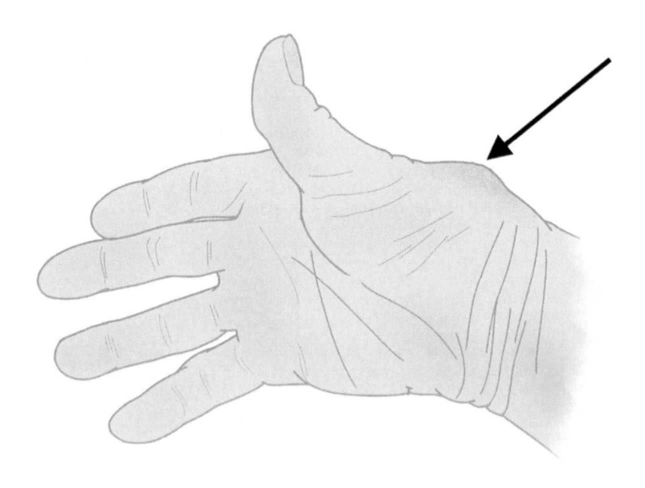

THUMB BASE ARTHRITIS DEFORMITY

☞ MIDDLE OF THE TOP SIDE (dorsum) OF THE WRIST:

A ganglion cyst, commonly a firm bump, ranging from the size of a pea to a grape, may occur around the middle of the back (dorsum) of the wrist. They are often noticed just incidentally and are not necessarily painful or tender to the touch. Ganglion cysts are true cysts that contain a gelatinous fluid rather than solid tissue. They can occur at any age and are not generally due to any injury or disease. In former times, they were treated by striking them with a large book or blunt object; this is not always necessary because sometimes they will break up or disappear on their own. If they do not, and especially if they cause any pain or discomfort, they can be reduced in size by draining the fluid contents under sterile conditions with a needle and syringe, but recurrence often occurs. The most reliable treatment is surgical removal. For many people with a ganglion cyst, the main concern is determining if the lump is a cancerous growth. This is easily determined by an experienced doctor.

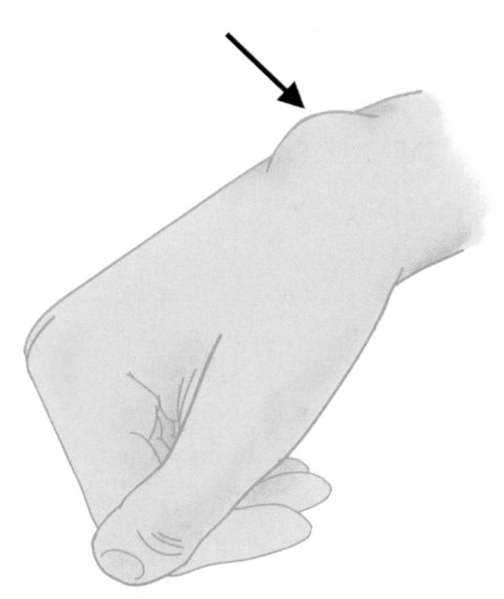

GANGLION CYST OF BACK OF WRIST

☞ GANGLION CYSTS IN OTHER LOCATIONS:

Ganglion cysts in locations other than the back side of the wrist are also fairly common, especially near the thumb on the palm side of the wrist and on the palm side of the finger. If they become painful or tender, they too can be drained with a needle and syringe in sterile conditions or be surgically removed.

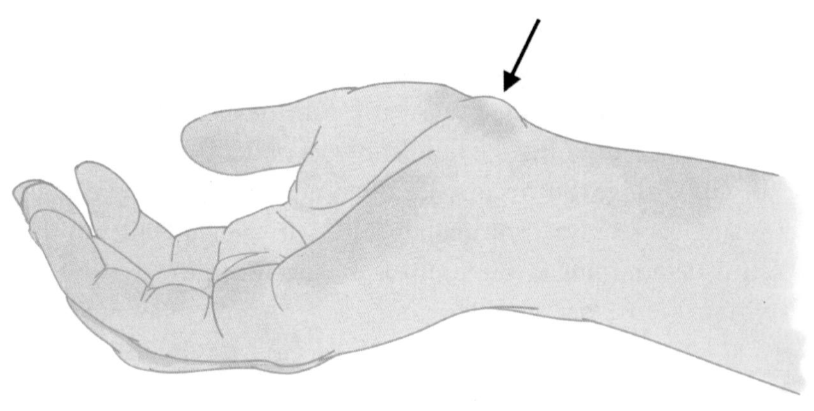

GANGLION CYST OF FRONT OF WRIST

☞ CORD-LIKE THICKENING OR NODULE IN THE PALM:

A thickening or nodule in the palm towards the small or ring finger (and sometimes other fingers or thumb) is more common in men of northern European heritage and is called Dupuytren's disease or contracture. Rather than a linear thickening, it may appear as a hard nodule. The condition tends to run in families, so a parent or relative might share the condition as well. Over time, the thickened cord may tend to draw the affected fingers into a clenched fist position, and as a result, it may become impossible to lay the hand flat on a surface. Stretching the fingers straight with a brace or physical therapy does not usually improve the contracture. Treatment becomes necessary when the inability to straighten the finger interferes with hand function by making it difficult to place the hand in a pocket or narrow space. The usual recommended treatment is surgical removal of the diseased tissue in the palm and/or finger (palmar fasciectomy). In selected cases, the cord may simply be cut rather than removed. This can be done either through a small puncture wound over the cord (percutaneous fasciotomy) or by first using an injected drug (collagenase clostridium histolyticum) into the cord to soften it, manipulating the finger into becoming straight. Recurrence of the contracture is more frequent with percutaneous fasciotomy or drug injection than with surgical removal.

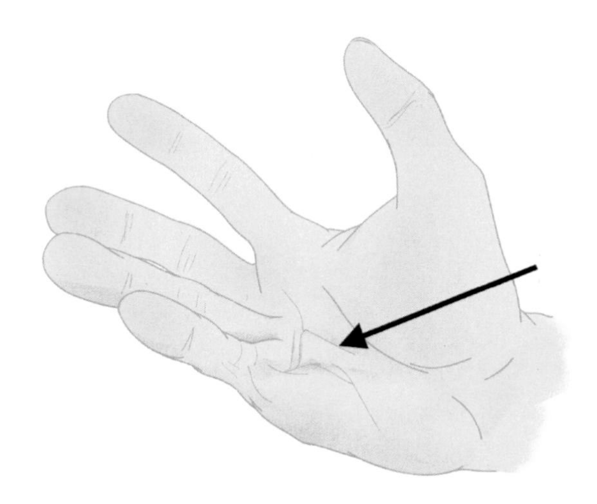

DUPUYTREN'S CONCRACTURE

☞ TUMORS IN ANY LOCATION OF THE HAND OR WRIST

Although much less common than any of the conditions mentioned above, a lump in the hand or wrist may be the result of either a benign or malignant (cancerous) tumor. A lump or bump that seems to be growing and enlarging, particularly if hard and not especially painful should raise suspicions of a tumor and should be brought to the attention of a doctor with specialized training in diseases of the hand and wrist.

Redness and Swelling

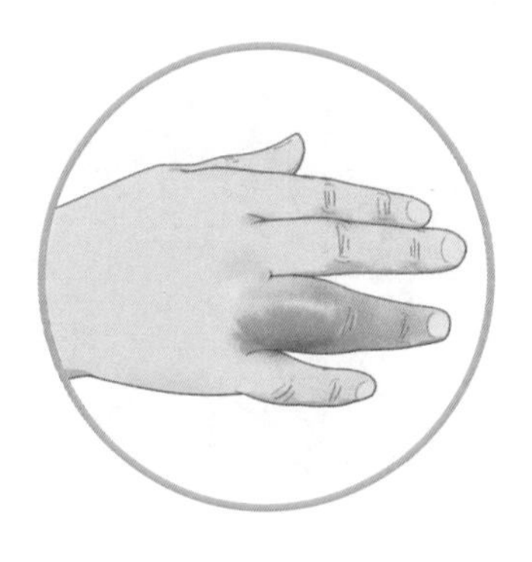

Redness and swelling are usually signs of inflammation. There may be many different causes for inflammation, but the most frequent is any of several types of arthritis or tendinitis.

Of the various causes of arthritis, the most common is "wear and tear" damage to a joint (osteoarthritis). Any joint in the hand and wrist can be affected by osteoarthritis, but it is especially common at the end joint of the fingers (distal interphalangeal joint) and the base of the thumb (as described in the "lumps and bumps" section). Wear and tear arthritis tends to affect older people and may tend to run in families. It can follow an old injury but as often occurs for no particular reason. When redness and swelling from osteoarthritis affects the wrist, it may be due to a past—often forgotten—sprain injury to the wrist ligaments, an unhealed bone fracture (navicular fracture), or degeneration of a bone (Keinbock's disease).

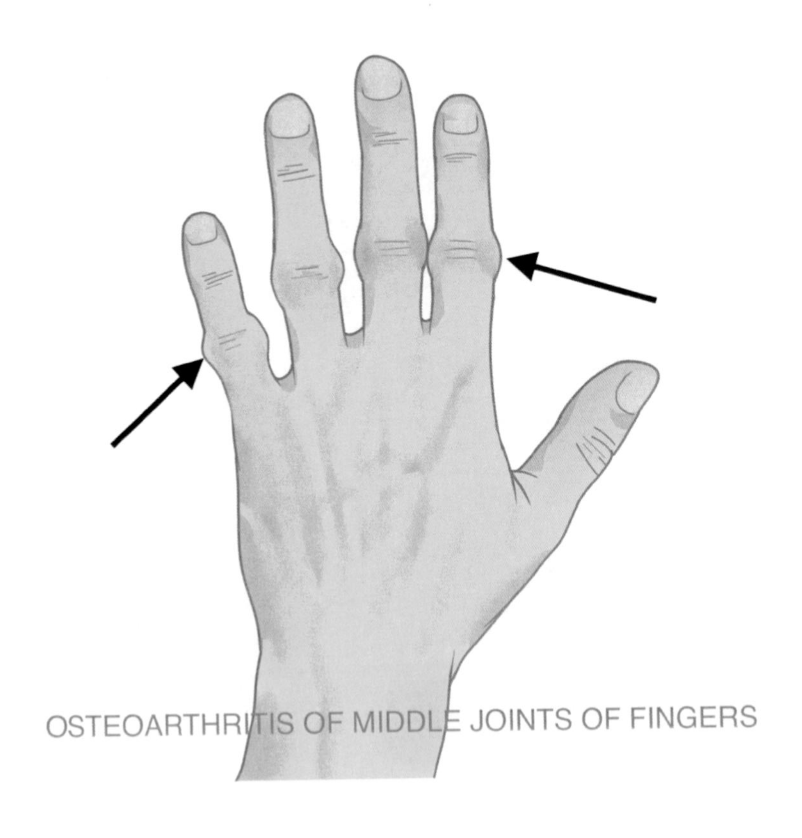

OSTEOARTHRITIS OF MIDDLE JOINTS OF FINGERS

There are, in addition to osteoarthritis, other possible causes of joint inflammation: an infection, rheumatoid disease, psoriasis, gout, pseudogout, lupus, Lyme disease, and other less common conditions.

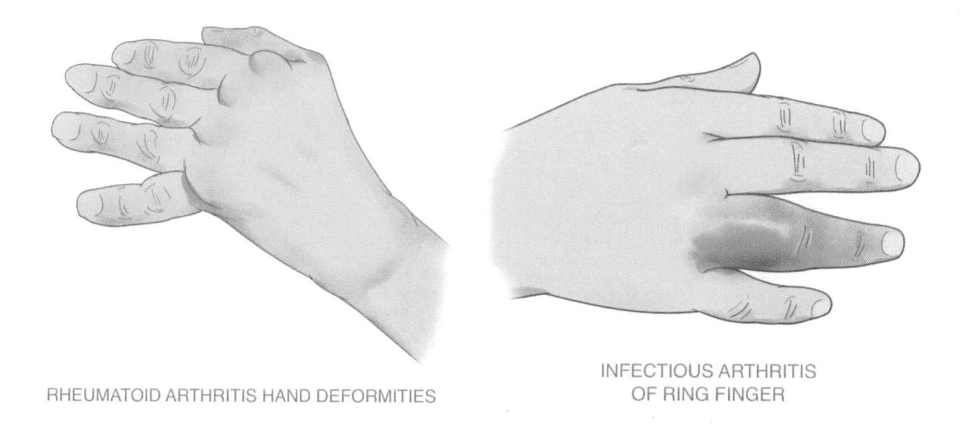

RHEUMATOID ARTHRITIS HAND DEFORMITIES

INFECTIOUS ARTHRITIS OF RING FINGER

Whatever the cause, arthritis of the involved joint is typically painful and tender to the touch, and results in some degree of stiffness of the finger or wrist. The appropriate treatment of arthritis depends mainly on the cause and the specific hand or wrist joint involved. In general, the initial treatment of the more common osteoarthritis with mild swelling, redness, and pain requires resting the involved joint and taking some form of non-steroidal anti-inflammatory medication (acetaminophen, aspirin, ibuprofen, naproxen, celecoxib, etc.). For the finger joints, rest may involve avoiding aggravating activity or wearing a finger splint to prevent movement of the involved joint. For the base of the thumb or wrist, resting the joint is most effectively accomplished by using a wrist brace that includes the base of the thumb. If finger stiffness becomes the major concern after the initial redness and swelling improves, gentle exercises with heat may be helpful.

The treatment of a type of arthritis that is not osteoarthritis should usually be directed by a medical professional and may involve specific prescription drugs, joint injections, physical or occupational therapy, or surgery. If the degree of redness, swelling, and pain is severe, arthritis due to infection or gout should be suspected. In such cases, urgent treatment by a medical professional should be sought.

Besides arthritis affecting the joints of the hand or wrist, redness and swelling may be due to inflammation of tendons (tendinitis), especially around the wrist. The most common forms of tendinitis are those described in the "Pain in the Hand and Wrist" section.

Pain in the Hand and Wrist

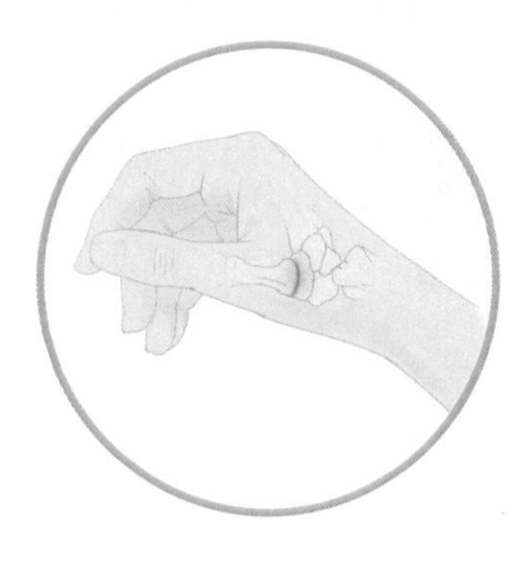

Painful problems in the hand and wrist are often due to many of the conditions described in the "Lumps and Bumps" and "Redness and Swelling" sections of this book. Sometimes, however, painful conditions arise that do not show a great deal of swelling, presenting more as sites of localized tenderness or pain in conjunction with motion of the fingers or wrist. Some of the more common causes of pain where swelling, redness, or a lump is not also seen include:

☞ **THE PALM SIDE OF ANY FINGER** may be painful due to inflammation of the tendons that pull the finger into the palm when making a fist (flexor tendinitis). Often, this occurs with a snapping or locking of the finger when grasping (trigger finger). The palm side of the finger may be tender particularly between the knuckle and middle joint (proximal interphalangeal joint) of the finger. This condition may be related to frequent repetitive motion (typing), diabetes, inflammatory diseases, or it may occur for no identifiable reason at all. If the finger is not snapping, or catching, or only rarely does so, it may improve by splinting the finger in a straight position at night and taking non-steroidal anti-inflammatory medication (acetaminophen, aspirin, naproxen, ibuprofen, celecoxib, etc.).

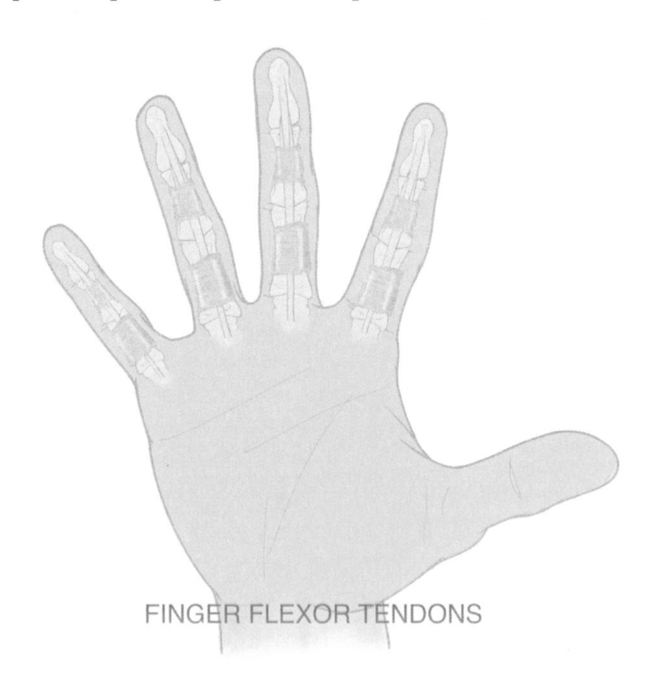

FINGER FLEXOR TENDONS

If these measures are not helpful, one should see a medical professional, who will very likely recommend a cortisone injection into the tissue sheath that surrounds the flexor tendons. If an injection is not helpful or if the condition recurs within a few weeks after an injection, surgery may be advised. The surgery usually involves enlarging the opening of the sheath that surrounds the flexor tendons using a local anesthetic, and is usually done without a hospital stay.

☞ **THE BASE OF THE THUMB** is a very frequent pain location, especially with pinching and grasping activities. There can be associated swelling or even a bony prominence, but it may be normal in appearance as well. It is due to "wear and tear" arthritis (osteoarthritis) and is more common in women and in people over the age of 60. The treatment of this condition is as described in the "Lumps and Bumps" section of this book and ranges from using a brace at night and for selected activities to injections or surgery.

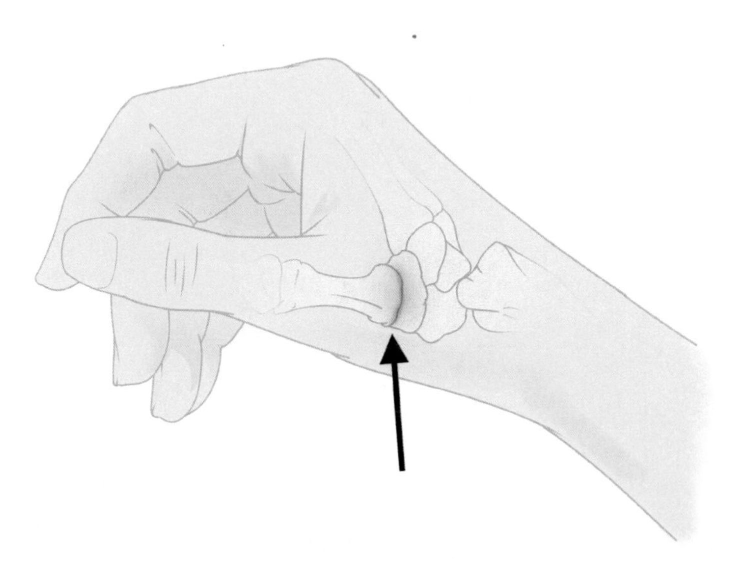

SITE OF PAIN WITH ARTHRITIS AT THUMB BASE

☞ **THE THUMB SIDE OF THE WRIST** is the site of a form of tendon irritation called DeQuervain's disease. It can be very painful and occurs with wrist motion or gripping. It may occur without any known cause, but some people experience it after unaccustomed repetitive wrist activity. It is usually accompanied with localized tenderness over the wrist bone about one inch from the base of the thumb. The usual initial treatment is immobilizing the wrist and thumb base by wearing a brace that supports the wrist and wraps around the thumb base (thumb shell splint), as well as a week or two of non-steroidal anti-inflammatory medication (acetaminophen, aspirin, naproxen, ibuprofen, celecoxib, etc.). If these measures do not improve the condition, examination by a medical professional is advised. The usual next treatment is an injection of cortisone into the involved tendon sheath at the wrist. If an injection is not successful or provides only temporary relief, surgery may be necessary.

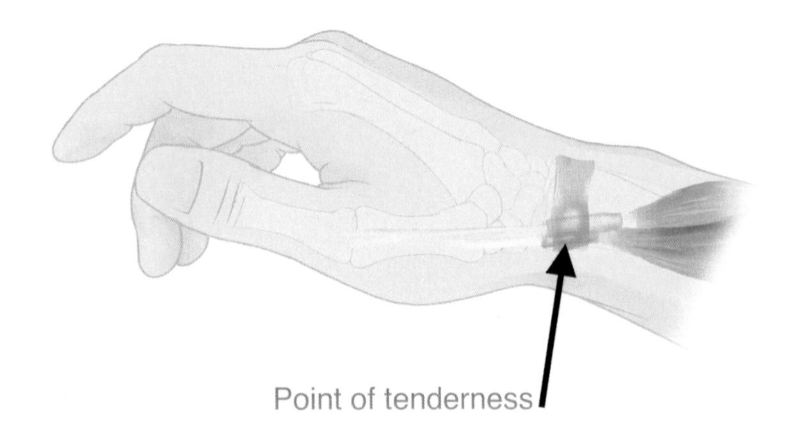

DeQuervain's Tendinitis

☞ **THE LITTLE FINGER SIDE OF THE WRIST** (ulnar) may also be the site of tendon irritation, but this is much less common than that of DeQuervain's disease on the thumb side. With this condition, pain is produced by bending wrist downward (flexion) and toward the thumb (radial deviation). Treatment usually involves resting the wrist with a support splint and non-steroidal anti-inflammatory mediation. If these measures fail, a cortisone injection into the involved tendon sheath may be necessary. Surgery is rarely required.

More commonly, pain on the little finger side of the wrist (ulnar) is due to "wear and tear" damage to the cartilage wafer (triangular fibrocartilage) that cushions the wrist bones (lunate and triquetrum) from the forearm bone (ulna). This may be due to a specific injury like a fall onto the outstretched wrist or to accumulated damage over time. There is usually localized tenderness on the top side (dorsum) of the wrist toward the little finger side.

Although an initial trial of using a wrist brace for few weeks may be helpful, most often, this condition requires an examination by a medical professional specializing in wrist and hand problems. The evaluation usually requires x-rays, and often, advanced imaging (MRI and/or CT scans). Depending on these studies, treatment may range from continued bracing to cortisone injections to arthroscopic or open surgery.

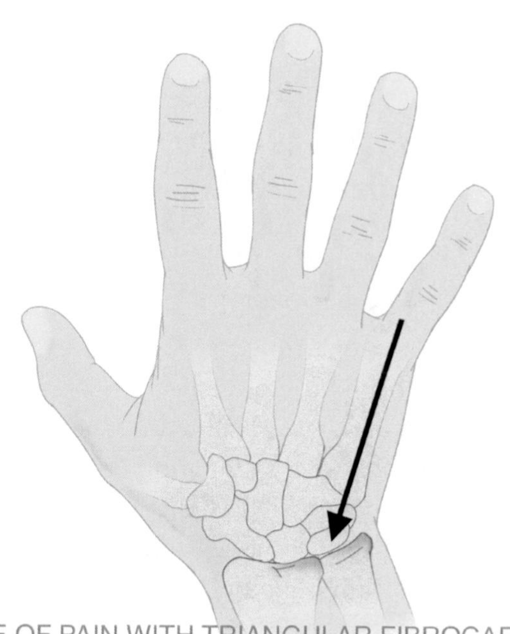

SITE OF PAIN WITH TRIANGULAR FIBROCARTILAGE INJURY

Another site of pain on the little finger side of the wrist is on the palm side and is due to either arthritis between two small wrist bones (pisiform and triquetrum) or an unrecognized fracture of another wrist bone (hamate), which is common in golfers. The diagnosis and treatment of either of these conditions is not in the realm of home treatment and requires an assessment by a specialized medical professional.

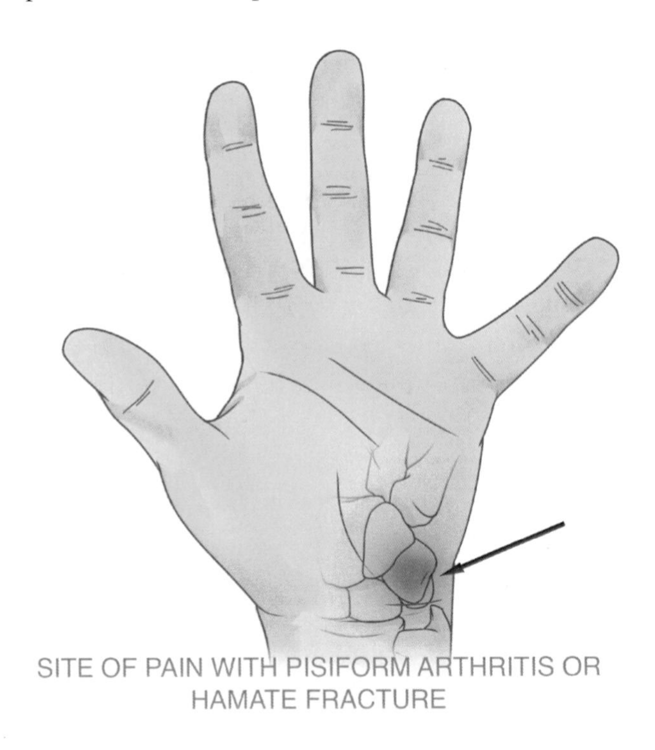

SITE OF PAIN WITH PISIFORM ARTHRITIS OR HAMATE FRACTURE

☞ **GENERALIZED PAIN IN THE WRIST**, neither thumb side nor little finger side, is often indicative of arthritic changes. Often this is due to an old, previously ignored, wrist injury to the ligaments, a broken bone (navicular), or degenerative changes to a small wrist bone (lunate; Keinbock's disease). Although the use of a wrist splint and non-steroidal anti-inflammatory medication may temporarily relieve the symptoms, treatment usually requires examination by a specialized medical professional. Surgical treatment will depend on the specific problem and extent of damage. It may include removing damaged bones (carpectomy), fusing together damaged joint surfaces (wrist fusion), or implanting an artificial wrist prosthesis (arthroplasty).

Numbness and Tingling

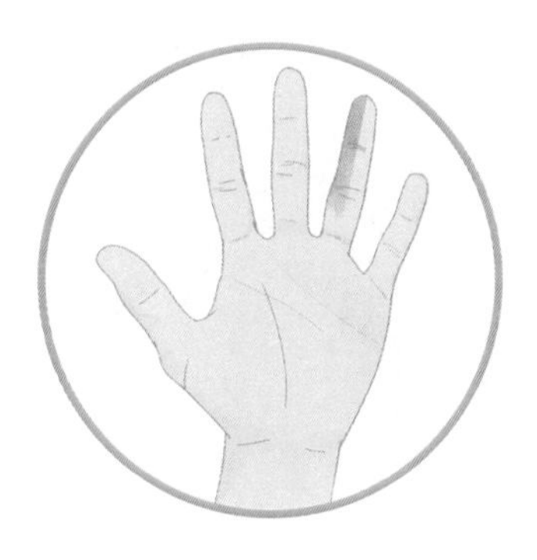

Numbness and Tingling of the hand extending into one or more fingers is a frequent complaint and is due, in most cases, to pressure on one of several nerves that supply feeling to various areas of the hand or arm. Even though the numbness and tingling may be in a finger or a portion of the hand, the site of nerve pressure or damage may be anywhere from the neck to the palm. The extent and location of the numbness or tingling usually is a good clue to what nerve is affected and where along the nerve the problem might be. Some of the more common problems where numbness and tingling is a prominent feature include:

☞ A SINGLE FINGER OR HALF OF A FINGER:

Feeling to the thumb and fingers is supplied by two tiny nerves (proper digital nerve) that run on the palmar side of the finger. Injury or pressure on the nerve can result in loss of feeling or tingling to that half of the finger or thumb.

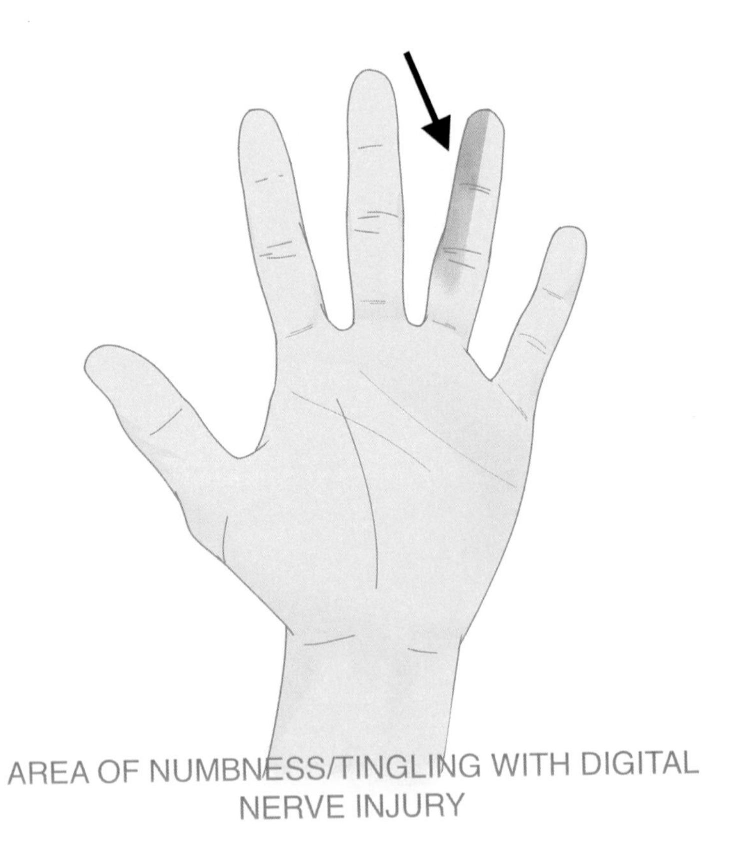

AREA OF NUMBNESS/TINGLING WITH DIGITAL NERVE INJURY

Although a deep cut to the finger that severs the nerve is the most common cause of numbness to half of the finger, anything that puts enough pressure on the proper digital nerve can produce tingling or numbness. This may be due to an adjacent cyst or bone spur, inflammation of the tendon sheath that lies beside the nerve, scarring that envelopes the nerve, or sometimes an excessively tight ring. The treatment for a severed nerve is surgical repair, and treatment for a compressed nerve is relief of the pressure on the nerve by surgical removal of the offending structure. A special problem that affects feeling over the inner half of the thumb is called bowler's thumb. This is due to repetitive pressure on the web side of the thumb due to such actions as poorly holding a bowling ball or excessive use of scissors or similar tools. The initial treatment for this condition is avoiding the offending activity or modifying what object is causing the excessive pressure.

☞ THE THUMB, INDEX, AND MIDDLE FINGER:

Undoubtedly, the most common complaint involving numbness and tingling in the hand is that of the thumb, index, middle, and sometimes half of the ring finger and is called carpal tunnel syndrome. It is caused by pressure on the nerve that supplies feeling to the palm side of the thumb, index, and middle fingers (median nerve) by a ligament (transverse carpal ligament) at the wrist. The symptoms are usually quite characteristic and include an increase in tingling at night while sleeping or while holding a steering wheel, newspaper, or book.

Any posture that places the wrist in a prolonged bent (flexed) position is apt to increase the tingling. The tingling can often be temporarily relieved by hanging one's hand down and shaking it. Over time the tingling symptoms might progress to loss of feeling or numbness and round-the-clock symptoms. Moreover, in severe cases, the palmar thumb muscles (thenar muscles) may begin wasting away, making fine-pinch activities difficult. Carpal tunnel syndrome can occur in either gender at any adult age, but it occurs most often in patients over age 40. It seems to occur most often in people who require repetitive wrist activity, but its relationship to specific jobs or hobbies is subject to debate.

The treatment is to relieve pressure on the median nerve at the wrist. In mild or early cases, especially when the only symptoms are at night while sleeping with few, if any, symptoms during daytime, the use of a wrist brace (cock-up splint), which prevents the wrist from falling into a bent position while sleeping, is all that is necessary. If symptoms persist despite the use of a nighttime splint, and particularly if symptoms occur during waking hours, then examination by a medical professional is advised. This examination may require additional tests (x-rays, ultrasound imaging, electrodiagnostic studies, etc.). The subsequent treatment might involve physical therapy, a cortisone injection into the palmar side of the wrist, or surgery to cut and lengthen the transverse carpal ligament. The latter might be accomplished by either a short incision in the palm near the wrist or an endoscope, with neither technique having a significantly better result.

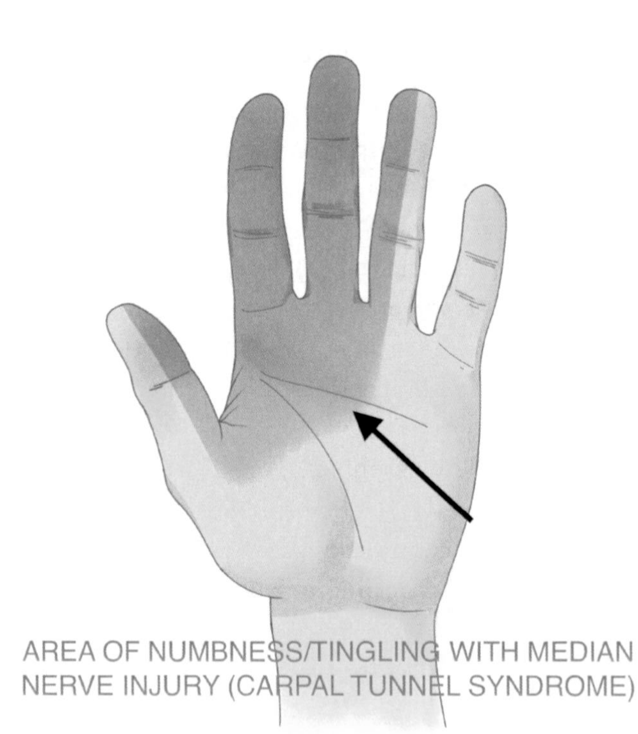

AREA OF NUMBNESS/TINGLING WITH MEDIAN NERVE INJURY (CARPAL TUNNEL SYNDROME)

Although rare in comparison with carpal tunnel syndrome, there can be other sites of median nerve compression that cause similar symptoms. One such site is just above the elbow where the median nerve can be compressed by a bone spur (supracondylar process) or a ligament (ligament of Struthers) that is present in as many as 13 percent of people. When the cause of the numbness and tingling is at the elbow, the symptoms do not have the characteristic nighttime and wrist position symptoms of carpal tunnel syndrome.

☞ THE PALM SIDE OF THE LITTLE AND RING FINGER:

Feeling to the little and half of the ring finger is supplied by the ulnar nerve, which enters the hand through a tunnel (Guyon's canal) similar to the carpal tunnel. Pressure on the ulnar nerve in Guyon's canal is very uncommon and is usually due to another structure within the canal crowding the nerve—for example, a ganglion cyst, a ballooning of a blood vessel (ulnar artery aneurysm), or a bone prominence. Treatment for Guyon's canal syndrome requires surgery to release the ligament that forms one side of the canal (volar carpal ligament) and remove any cyst or additional abnormal mass taking up space within the canal.

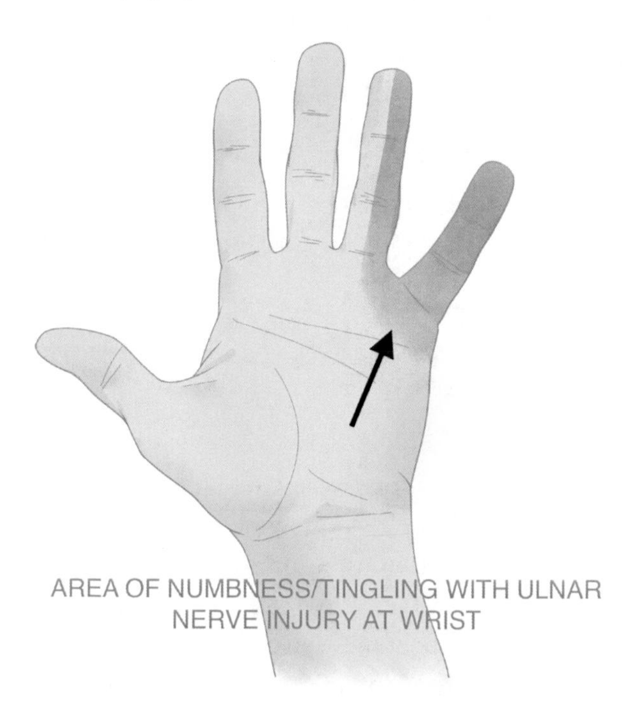

AREA OF NUMBNESS/TINGLING WITH ULNAR NERVE INJURY AT WRIST

☞ BOTH THE PALM AND TOP SIDE OF THE LITTLE AND RING FINGER:

Much more common than pressure on the ulnar nerve at the wrist (Guyon's canal syndrome) is pressure on the ulnar nerve at the elbow, the so-called funny bone. This condition is called cubital tunnel syndrome and results in numbness and tingling in the little and half of the ring finger on both the palm and top sides, as well as on the back of the hand above the little and ring finger. In addition, it frequently causes weakness and wasting of the small muscles of the hand that control side-to-side motion of the fingers and pinch.

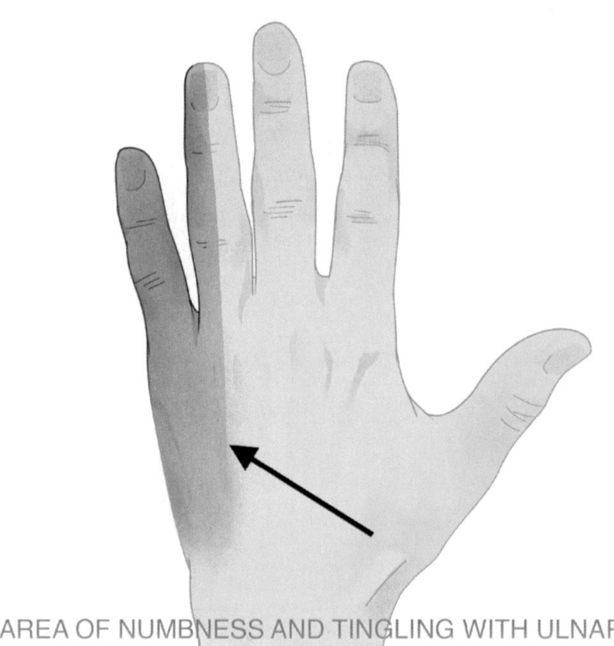

AREA OF NUMBNESS AND TINGLING WITH ULNAR NERVE INJURY AT ELBOW

When cubital tunnel syndrome is relatively mild, the tingling and numbness just occur when holding the elbow in a fully bent position. As it becomes more severe, the symptoms become continuous and muscle-wasting becomes obvious. The treatment for intermittent, mild symptoms usually starts with the use of a brace at night, which prevents the elbow from being fully bent. However, more severe and continuous symptoms of numbness and tingling require fairly urgent treatment, since neglect can result in irreversible wasting away of the small muscles of the hand that control dexterity and pinch. The appropriate treatment requires surgery to relieve the pressure and entrapment of the ulnar nerve as it passes behind the funny bone (medial epicondyle). In more severe cases, the surgery might also include gently shifting the location of the ulnar nerve from behind the elbow to in front of the elbow (ulnar nerve anterior transposition).

☞ BACK OF THE HAND ON THE THUMB SIDE:

Feeling on the back of the hand on the thumb side as well as most of the top of the thumb, index, and middle finger is supplied by the superficial radial nerve. This nerve passes from the back of the forearm to the wrist and hand just under the skin. Because it is so close to the surface of the skin at the wrist where little tissue padding exists, the nerve can be subject to compression and injury from, for example, a tight watch-band, bracelet, or anything tight wrapping the wrist such as a water ski towrope or handcuffs. The nerve can also be injured by a deep cut over the thumb side of the wrist or by surgery for the base of the thumb. In addition, though not very common, it can be pinched by a wrist tendon as it emerges from the forearm to the wrist (Wartenberg's syndrome). Often, in addition to numbness and tingling, many people with compression of the superficial radial nerve complain of annoying sensitivity to touch (allodynia) on the thumb side of the back of the hand and wrist.

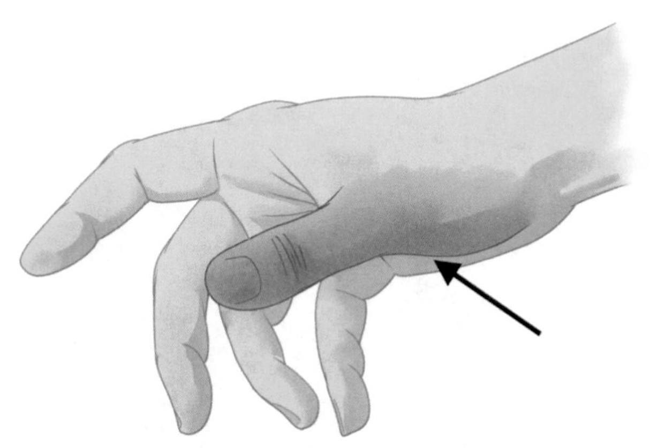

AREA OF NUMBNESS/TINGLING WITH SUPERFICIAL RADIAL NERVE INJURY

The treatment of superficial radial nerve compression depends on the cause. When the condition is due to ongoing compression from a tight band or a sudden pull from a rope around the wrist, often it will improve with time, and treatment is unnecessary. When painful sensitivity is the chief concern, various forms of desensetization can be effective, like gently rubbing the sensitive area of the hand with objects of various textures. In the rare instance of a medical professional diagnosing Wartenberg's syndrome, the treatment requires surgery to lengthen the tendon compressing the nerve.

☞ THE ARM OR FOREARM THAT EXTENDS TO THE HAND:

Feeling that involves the arm or forearm and includes the hand is supplied by nerves that are at the neck (cervical nerve roots) or shoulder (brachial plexus). Numbness or tingling that affects the hand or fingers but also includes portions of the arm or forearm should suggest that the problem is arising at the neck or shoulder area. Treatment for these conditions should be left to a doctor with special training for dealing with nerve and spine problems. If there is accompanying muscle weakness in the hand or arm, appropriate treatment assumes greater urgency.

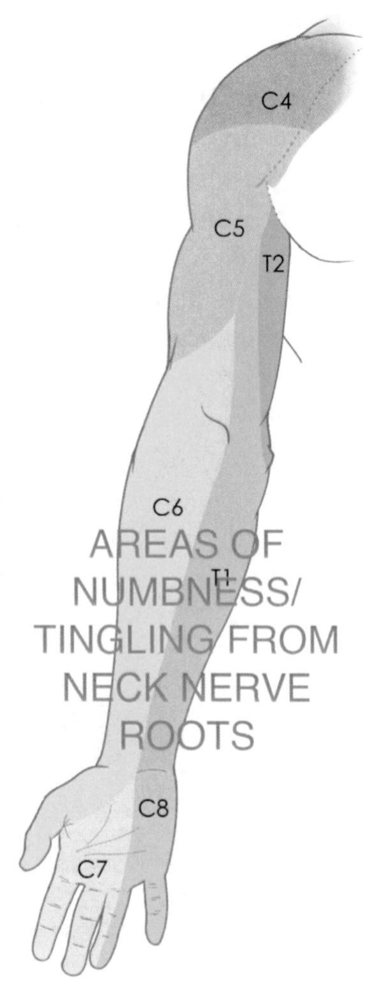

AREAS OF NUMBNESS/ TINGLING FROM NECK NERVE ROOTS

Circulation and Color Changes

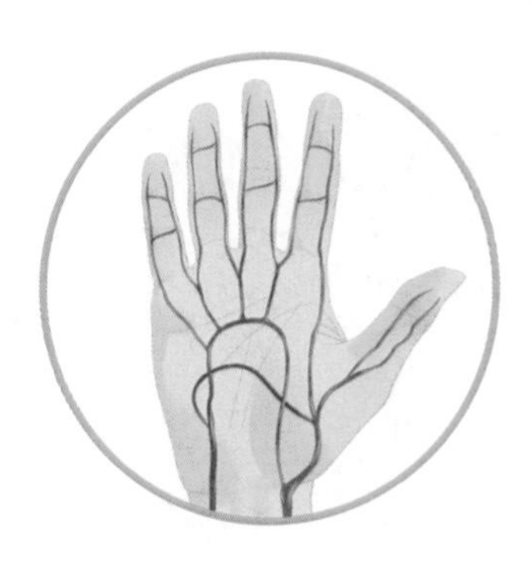

Adequate circulation of blood to the hand is extremely important. Blood normally flows to the hand through two major arteries at the wrist (radial and ulnar arteries) and then continues to the fingers through two smaller arteries to each finger (proper digital arteries). Between all these blood vessels there are many branches that connect to each other. These connecting branches usually ensure that there is adequate circulation to the hand and fingers even if one artery is completely injured or blocked due to a blood vessel disease (atherosclerosis or arteritis).

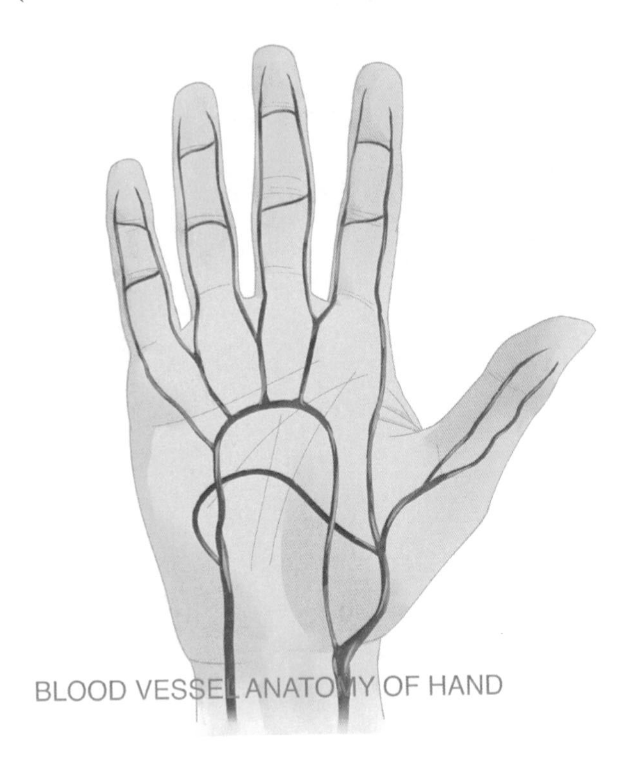
BLOOD VESSEL ANATOMY OF HAND

If circulation to the hand or finger is partially impaired, the finger might become painful and pale in color with exposure to cold temperatures or if one consumes caffeine or nicotine. Partial impairment of circulation to the fingers might occur if one of the two major arteries at the wrist (radial or ulnar arteries) becomes blocked and there are not enough connecting branches between them. A common cause of ulnar artery blockage at the wrist is repetitive blunt injury to the base of the palm on the little finger side (hypothenar hammer syndrome). This may occur when one pounds the wrist against something stationary like a stuck door or drawer. Radial artery blockage is now increasingly seen as a result of a medical procedure when a blood vessel catheter is placed into the radial artery at the wrist for certain heart operations or for monitoring a patient in a life-threatening situation in an intensive care unit.

If there is severe blood vessel injury involving several arteries or extensive blood vessel blockage by disease, there may be insufficient circulation to the fingers to nourish the tissues. In such cases, finger ulcers or gangrene of one or several fingers may result, necessitating urgent medical care.

The treatment of inadequate circulation to the hand or fingers depends on the severity of the situation. If mild and without the development of ulceration sores, protection from cold and the avoidance of nicotine or caffeine may be all that is necessary. If more severe, medications to improve blood flow or surgery to bypass or reconstruct a blocked artery may be advised. If gangrene has occurred, amputation may be required.

A somewhat common circulation problem affecting the fingers is the temporary loss of finger blood-flow due to the arteries in the fingers going into spasm in response to certain stimuli. The stimulus is most often exposure to cold but may also be exposure to caffeine, nicotine, or even simple stress. After a short period of time, the blood vessels relax and blood flow to the fingertip returns. As blood flow resumes, the fingertip color changes from white or pale to bluish-dark and then normal color. This condition is called Raynaud's phenomenon, and is not caused by any disease that permanently block the blood vessels and does not result in finger ulcers or gangrene. Treatment of Raynaud's phenomenon is usually not necessary, but if it occurs with such frequency that it interferes with work or outdoor activities, medications to make the blood vessels less sensitive to spasm may be helpful.

If Raynaud's phenomenon is occurring along with blood vessel disease (atherosclerosis or arteritis) it can eventually lead to non-healing ulcers or gangrene. When this is the case, it is called Raynaud's disease and may be associated with other serious diseases (lupus or scleroderma).

Although quite rare, circulation problems in the hand can be a result of an abnormal formation of blood vessels from birth or a tumor of abnormal blood vessels. These conditions can cause either a lack of blood flow to parts of the hand or fingers or give rise to clots, which plug blood vessels in the fingers. Abnormal blood vessel formations can also cause excessive blood flow, which, in a child, can lead to overgrowth of parts of the hand or fingers. Treatment of this condition is dependent on how much of a problem the malformation is causing. It can sometimes be treated by injecting, under x-ray control, small bead-like particles to block the main feeding blood vessels, decreasing blood flow. In other cases it can be treated by surgical removal of all or some of the feeding blood vessels. However, even with surgical removal, recurrence of the problem is common.

Stiffness and Loss of Movement

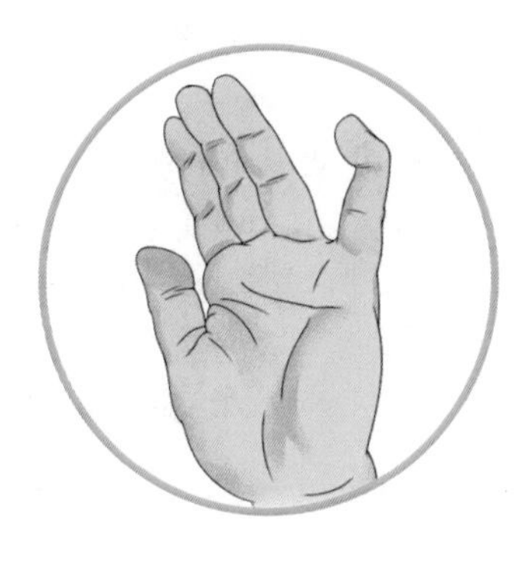

Loss of movement of the hand and fingers can be caused by several different problems—paralyzed muscles, stiff or frozen joints, or tendon disruption. Nerve injury or disease can paralyze or weaken the muscles that are responsible for producing movement. Arthritis or injuries of the joints of the fingers or wrist can limit motion or stiffen the joint completely. Tendons that connect muscles to the joints can be either cut or ruptured, which makes the muscles unable to move the wrist or finger.

☞ NERVE INJURY:

There are many nerves that travel to the wrist and hand, and most provide both feeling and muscle movement. Nerve problems that affect the feeling function (sensibility or sensation) have largely been discussed in the "Numbness and Tingling" section. There are three major nerves that serve the muscles, providing movement for the hand and wrist: the median, ulnar, and radial nerves. These can be injured or diseased at any location from the neck to the forearm and hand.

- The median nerve is responsible for serving some of the muscles that bend the wrist (flexion) and move the fingers in the direction of making a fist (finger flexion), as well as some of the muscles that move the thumb. Therefore, problems of the median nerve result in an inability to grasp and a weakness of pinch.
- The ulnar nerve serves some of the muscles that bend the wrist and the little and ring fingers (flexion), and the small muscles of the hand, which spread the fingers apart and help control the thumb. Problems of the ulnar nerve result in a clumsy hand that is unable to do fine activities.
- The radial nerve supplies all the muscles that lift the wrist (extension) and straighten the fingers and thumb. Problems of the radial nerve produce a drop wrist, drooping fingers, and a thumb-in-palm posture.

The treatment of any nerve injury is much the same. If a nerve is cut or torn and it is treated within a year or two of the injury, it should be surgically repaired or reconstructed with a nerve graft. If a nerve injury is seen quite late, the function of the paralyzed muscles can sometimes be substituted through a surgery that attaches a less important muscle to the paralyzed muscle tendon (tendon transfer).

☞ STIFF OR FROZEN JOINTS:

Limited motion of joints can occur for a variety of reasons. Arthritis, as discussed in the "Redness and Swelling" section, is a very common cause, especially in older people. Direct injury to a joint from a severe sprain or a blunt blow may damage the joint surface or cause a bone fracture, which interferes with the ability of a joint to easily move through its normal range. Simply immobilizing a joint for a long period of time in a cast or splint can cause the joint to stiffen.

The treatment of a stiff or frozen joint, when the joint surfaces are not severely damaged, usually involves therapy to stretch the joint back to its normal amount of motion. This is often best accomplished under the supervision of a trained therapist. It may also require the prolonged use of an appropriate splint or brace to stretch the joint or hold it in a corrected position. If therapy and/or splints are not sufficient to restore adequate motion of the joint, surgery to release the tightened envelope (capsule) surrounding the joint may be advised (capsulectomy), followed by continued therapy. In patients with severe damage to the surface of the joint, attempts to stretch the joint are usually unsuccessful. In such cases, surgically cutting out the joint and replacing it with an artificial joint or a piece of the patient's own tendon or soft tissue (arthroplasty) may be necessary to restore some amount of functional motion.

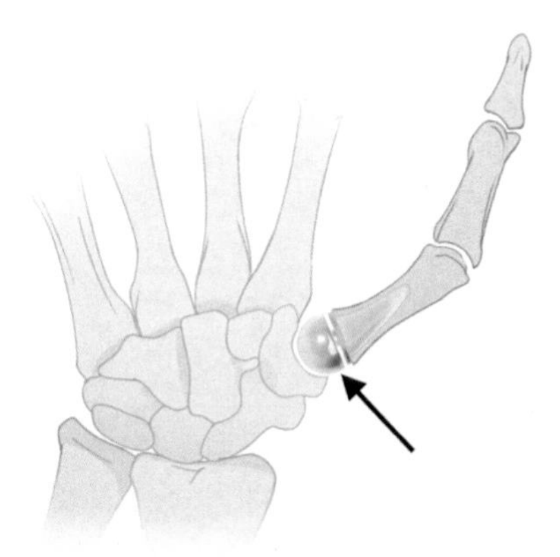

BASE OF THUMB ARTICIAL JOINT REPLACMENT

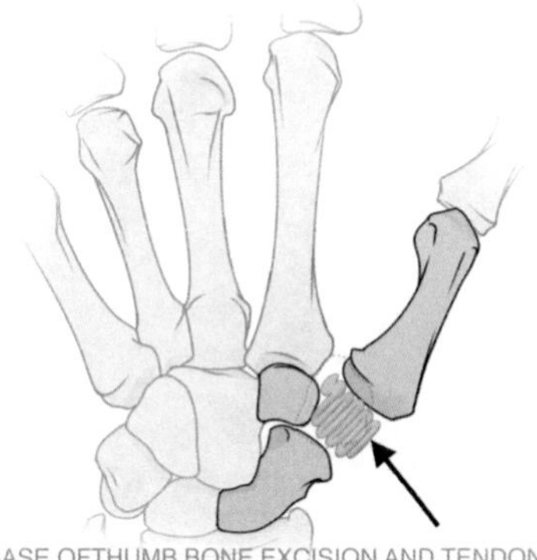

BASE OFTHUMB BONE EXCISION AND TENDON REPLACEMENT

☞ CUT TENDON:

Tendons are the rope-like structures that connect a muscle to a bone across a joint that produces movement of a joint. A tendon can be cut by a penetrating injury, like a knife or saw cut, or in some cases rupture from a forceful movement or degeneration of the tendon strength. When a tendon is disrupted, whatever the cause, it is unable to produce any movement to a joint. Any tendon can be damaged, but the most common problems are in:

- The tendon(s) that bend (flexion) a finger or thumb as result of a deep cut over the palm side of a finger, thumb, or palm;
- The tendons that bend (flexion) several fingers and thumb with a deep cut over the palm side of the wrist; and
- The tendons that straighten the fingers with a cut over the knuckle joints or over the back of the hand.

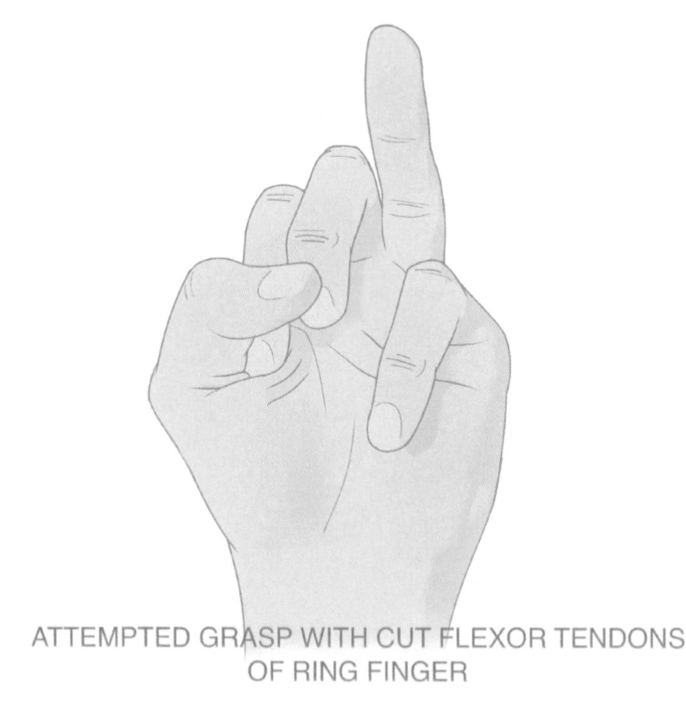

ATTEMPTED GRASP WITH CUT FLEXOR TENDONS OF RING FINGER

☞ RUPTURED TENDON:

Tendon ruptures that do not involve a penetrating injury can occur as result of a sudden forced movement. The most common examples of these are:

- A rupture of the tendon that straightens the end joint of the finger is called a "mallet finger". This injury is usually a result of a bending force (flexion) on the tip of a finger while holding it in a straight position (extension). This injury might occur with surprisingly little force. The resulting deformity is a droop of the fingertip at the end joint and an inability to straighten the fingertip. The ruptured tendon end might also include a small fragment of bone. Treatment of this condition usually requires immobilizing the finger in a fully straight position with a finger splint for several weeks. If the injury is seen after several weeks or if an associated large fragment of bone is also injured, surgery to reattach the tendon or attached bone fragment may be necessary.

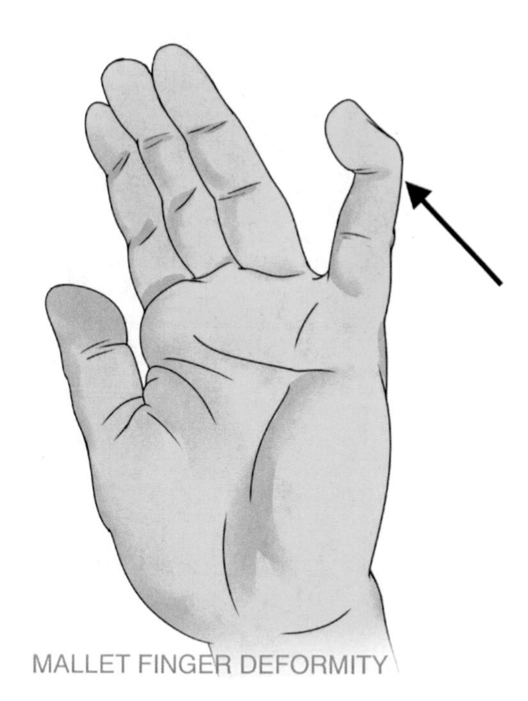

MALLET FINGER DEFORMITY

- A rupture of the tendon that straightens the middle joint of the finger (extensor tendon) is called a boutonniere deformity. This injury is usually a result of a strong bending force to the finger while it is held in a straight position. With this tendon rupture, there is an inability to straighten the middle joint of the finger. Treatment of this condition, if seen within a few days of the injury, may be successful by simply splinting the middle joint of the finger in a fully straight position. However, this does require full-time splinting for as long as six to eight weeks. Unfortunately, many times, the diagnosis of a boutonniere deformity is not made until several weeks after the injury, and in such cases, surgery by a specialized medical professional is often necessary. If untreated or if initial treatment is not successful, a permanent bend (flexion contracture) in the finger middle joint is the end result.

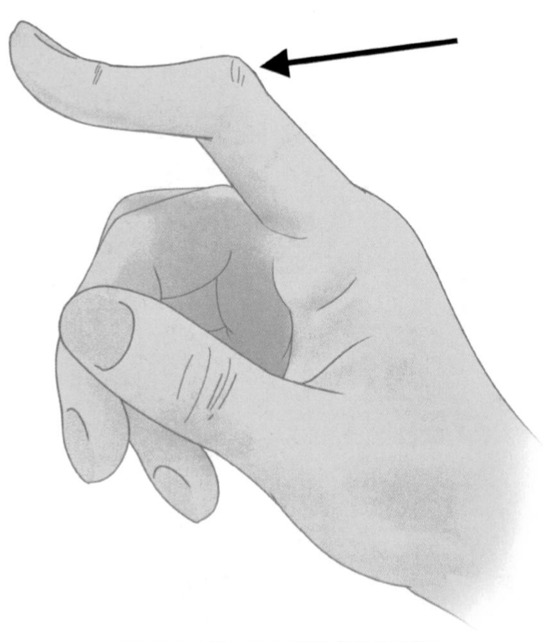

BOUTONNIERE DEFORMITY

- A rupture of the tendon that bends (flexion) the end joint of the finger (flexor profundus tendon) is called a football jersey finger. This injury is caused by a forced straightening of the finger end joint while it is held bent in a strenuous grasping activity. As the name implies, the injury is most common in young football or rugby athletes when a defender unsuccessfully grasps onto an opponent's jersey. With this tendon rupture, there is an inability to bend the end joint of the finger. Treatment of this injury mandates surgery to reattach the flexor tendon to the end of the finger. If treatment is delayed beyond a few weeks, reattachment may not be possible because the tendon retracts into the palm. In such cases, a more complex surgery requiring a tendon graft may be necessary.

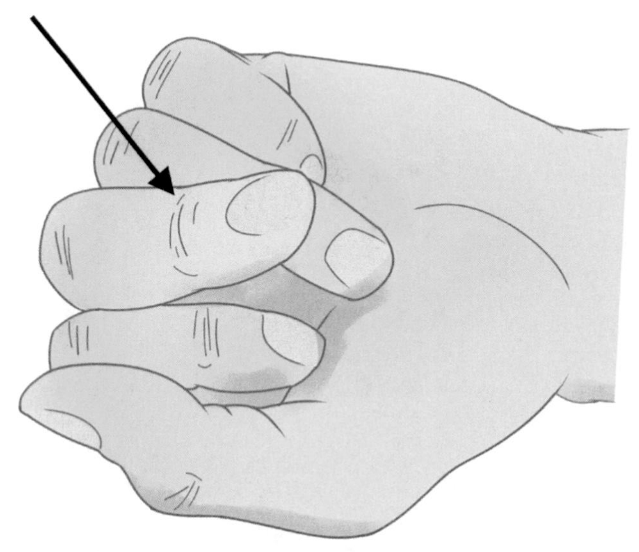

JERSEY FINGER INJURY TO MIDDLE FINGER

Snapping or Clicking Movements

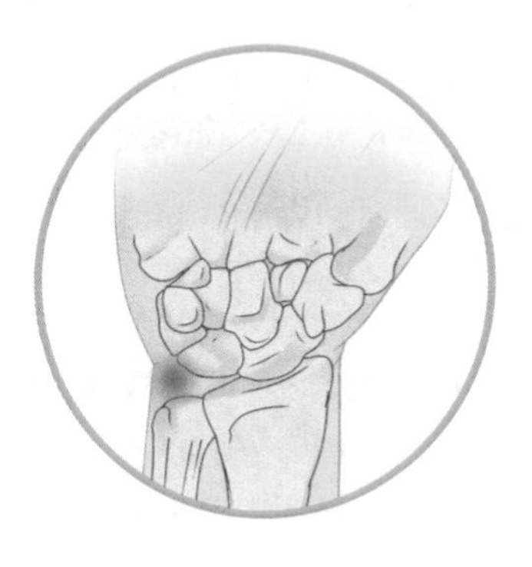

☞ FINGER OR THUMB SNAPPING OR CLICKING:

Snapping or clicking movements are usually due to either a tendon problem or ligament laxity, which results in abnormal catching or clunking movements. There are a few somewhat common conditions that can cause this to occur.

- **TRIGGER THUMB OR FINGER:**

  By far the most common cause of a snapping movement of the thumb or a finger is due to a restriction of the normal smooth gliding of the thumb or finger flexor tendon. The flexor tendon is held in place by a series of strong fibrous bands called pulleys, which form a sheath or tunnel through which the tendon passes. If there is any condition that causes a thickening of the pulleys or an enlargement of the tendon, the tendon cannot easily glide through its sheath and must instead shimmy or force its way through the sheath. This is most commonly due to inflammation about the tendon that can cause either scarring of the pulleys or swelling of the tendon.

  In most cases, the snapping seems to start for no apparent reason, but it may begin following prolonged repetitive grasping activities. It is more common in people with diabetes or inflammatory disorders like rheumatoid disease. In severe cases, the finger may actually lock in a bent position and require manipulation to be unlocked. It may or may not be painful.

  The treatment of trigger finger depends on how severe the problem is and how long it has been present. If the snapping has been only occasional and has been a problem for only a short time, especially if it occurs only after awakening, simply immobilizing the finger in a straight position with a splint at night while sleeping may be effective treatment. If it occurs more frequently during the day and has been present for several months, treatment by a medical professional is usually necessary. In this case, the initial treatment will most likely be an injection of cortisone into the tendon sheath. This may be done in conjunction with part time splinting and physical therapy. If one or more injections do not cure the condition, surgery may be recommended to enlarge the opening of the tendon sheath.

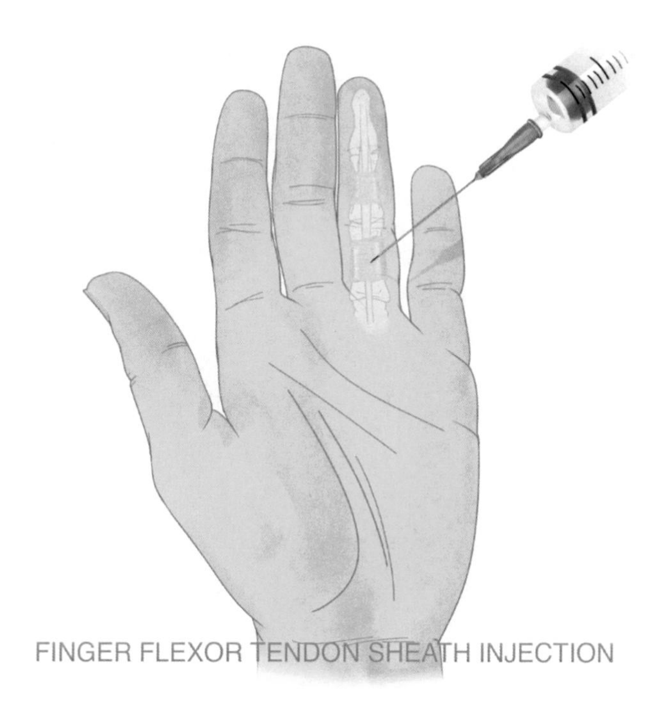

FINGER FLEXOR TENDON SHEATH INJECTION

- A much less common cause of finger snapping, which is often confused with trigger finger, is instability of the tendon that straightens the finger (extensor tendon) over the knuckle joint. This condition is usually a result of an injury to the ligaments that hold the extensor tendon in place over the top of the knuckle, and most often occurs in the middle finger. The injury is usually the result of a direct blow over the knuckle from a fall or punch. With this condition, a snapping sensation is felt over the top of the knuckle (usually middle finger) with making a fist and with straightening the finger. Initially, the snapping is painful, but over time it may become painless though still annoying. The treatment of this condition is usually surgical repair of the torn ligament, but if seen early, the use of a specialized splint to hold the knuckle joint is a fully straight position for several weeks may be effective.

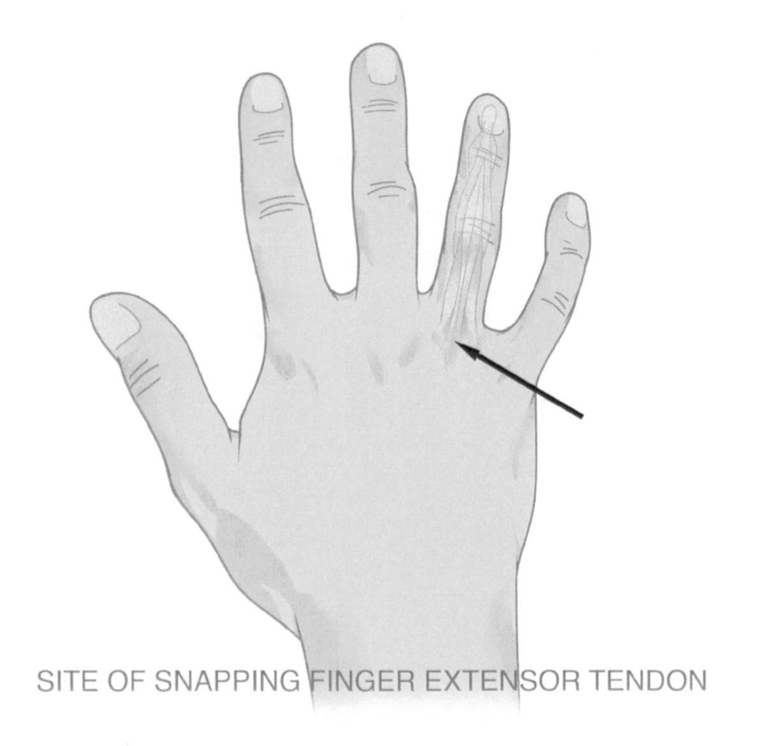
SITE OF SNAPPING FINGER EXTENSOR TENDON

- Another cause of a snapping or catching sensation of a finger may be due to a ligament injury (collateral ligament) to either the knuckle or middle joint of the finger that fails to heal normally. The collateral ligaments of the finger joints function to maintain the joint in proper alignment as it moves through its full range of motion. As a result of a sprain injury to a finger joint, the collateral ligament may be torn to a degree that it can no longer provide sufficient joint stability. When this occurs, the joint can seem to jump or click rather than smoothly glide as it moves. This condition may be painful but is often more of a cause of annoying discomfort. If the accompanying discomfort becomes a sufficient enough problem, surgical repair may be warranted. The surgery involves tightening the ligament by re-attaching it to its proper position at its location of injury. Even with repair, some amount of residual joint stiffness is not unusual.

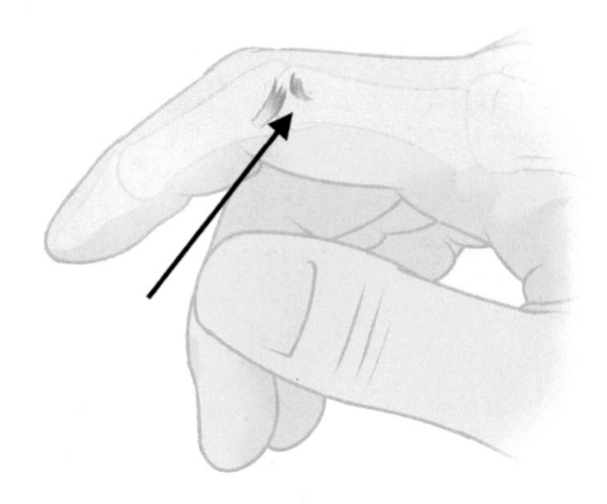

RUPTURED FINGER JOINT COLLATERAL LIGAMENT

☞ SNAPPING OR CLICKING OF THE WRIST:

There are several causes for the wrist to have a snapping sensation, or what is more typically described as a clunking sensation. The wrist joint is actually a collection of 8 separate bones plus 2 forearm bones, and rather than consisting of a single joint, it includes multiple joints between those 10 bones, which, acting together, function as a single universal joint.

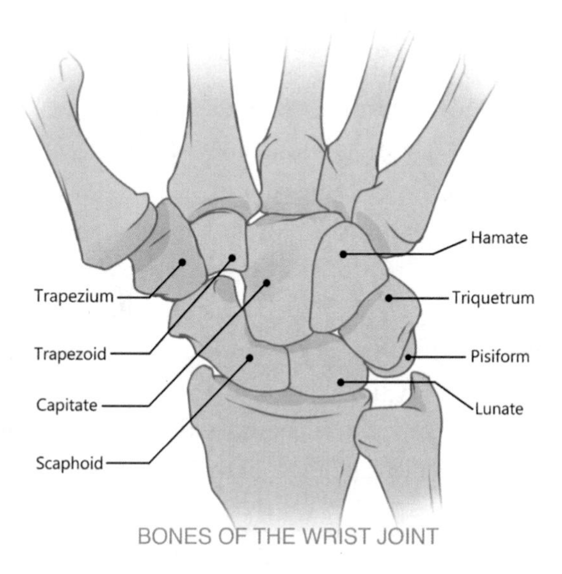

BONES OF THE WRIST JOINT

For this arrangement to work properly, these 10 bones must be linked by normally functioning ligaments to maintain the proper position of each small bone as the wrist moves up and down, side to side, and rotates palm up and palm down. Injury to any of these ligaments can occur, especially, by a fall onto the outstretched hand and wrist.

- If the force of the injury is sufficient enough to completely tear a ligament, and if it does not heal with its normal strength, then the teamwork between the multiple small wrist bones becomes disturbed. When this occurs, a distinct, painful clunking sensation may occur with wrist motion. This condition is called traumatic wrist instability. The diagnosis of this condition usually requires an assessment by a medical professional with special training in wrist problems. X-rays and, often, special imaging (MRI or CT Scans) or even arthroscopic examination is necessary to evaluate the specific ligament injury. Treatment usually requires surgery to repair or reconstruct the injured ligament(s) or fuse together the unstable bones.

- Another cause of wrist "clunking" can be unrelated to any wrist injury, but due to an excessive amount of wrist ligament laxity that a person may be born with. This condition is commonly called joint hypermobility syndrome or carpal instability nondissociative (CIND). Individuals with this problem can, at will, produce a "clunk" (usually painless) with a visible distortion of the wrist's appearance. This condition is more common in women and may be associated with certain diseases (Ehlers-Danlos Syndrome; Marfan's Syndrome). Carpal instability nondissociative may not be especially disabling and in such cases may not require treatment. However, when it is associated with considerable wrist weakness and interferes with activity, protective bracing and strengthening of the wrist muscles (extensor carpi ulnaris) or specific proprioceptive therapy may be advised. In severe instances or when bracing and therapy are not effective, surgery to tighten the lax wrist ligaments (wrist ligament plication) or fusion of a portion of the wrist bones may be necessary.

- Injury or degeneration of the cartilage wafer (triangular fibrocartilage) that cushions the end of the forearm bone (ulna) from the wrist bones (triquetrum and lunate) may be another cause of snapping or clicking of the wrist, as discussed in the "Pain and Tenderness" section. Usually with this condition, the symptoms are more described as grating sensation and pain that coincides with forearm rotation or wrist deviation towards the little finger direction. Diagnosis and treatment for triangular fibrocartilage injuries is as described in the "Pain and Tenderness" section.

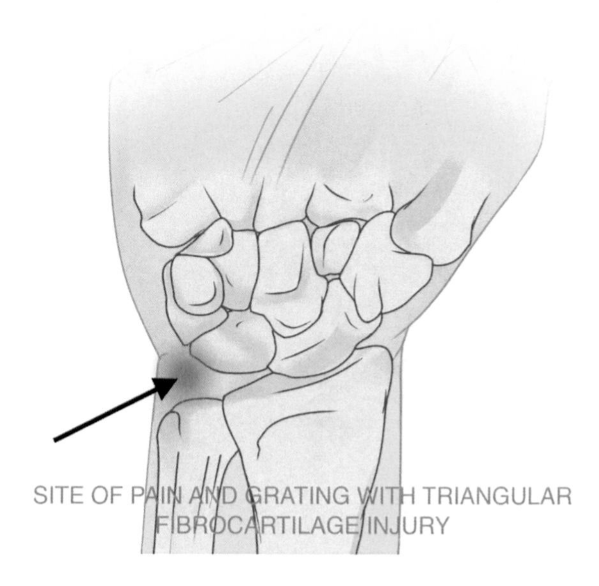

Deformity

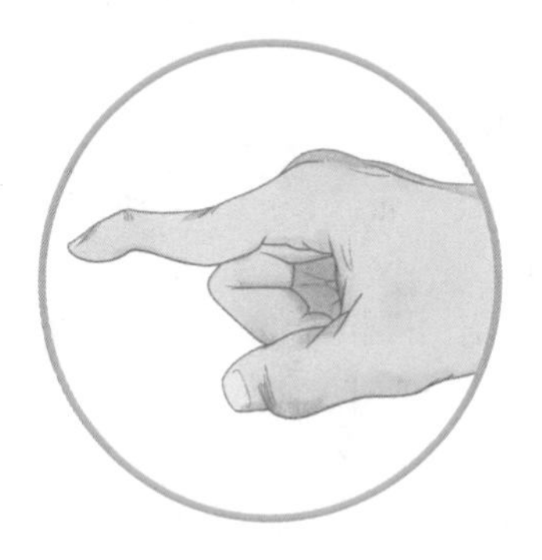

Many of the common deformities of the hand and wrist have been described in other sections but deserve mention as deformities, as well. These include deformities resulting from arthritis, tendon injury, or poorly healed fractures, and include:

☞ HEBERDEN'S NODE:

As described in the "Lumps and Bumps" section, this is a bony enlargement of the end joint (distal interphalangeal joint) of the finger. It is due to wear and tear arthritis (osteoarthritis). Treatment is as described on page 4.

☞ BOUCHARD'S NODE:

This is a bony enlargement of the finger middle joint (proximal interphalangeal joint) and usually causes a bend (flexion contracture) in the middle joint, which makes it difficult to fully straighten the finger. In many regards, a Bouchard's node is similar to a Heberden's node but in a different joint. However, unlike a Heberden's node, a joint with a Bouchard's node is frequently painful. It is due to arthritis.

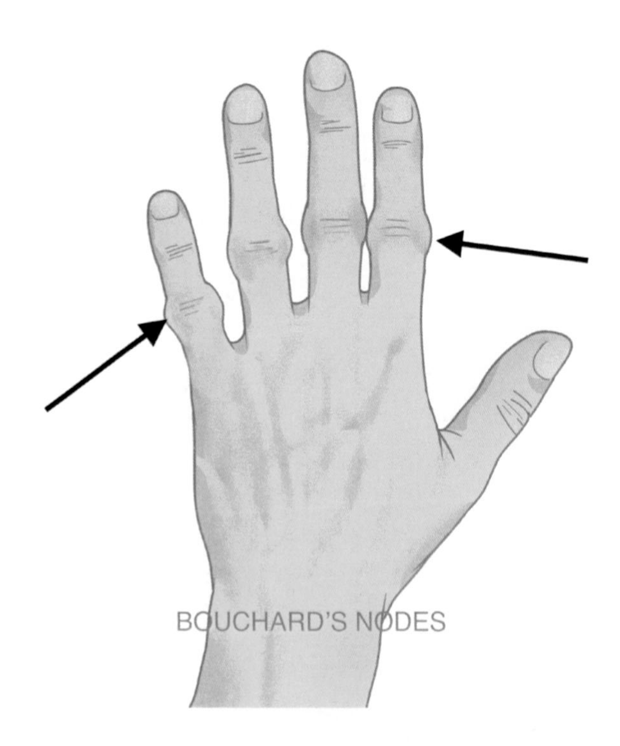

BOUCHARD'S NODES

Treatment depends mainly on how disabling the condition is in terms of pain or stiffness. If symptoms are relatively mild with occasional pain and only minimal flexion deformity, then home treatment of periodic splinting, non-steroidal anti-inflammatory medications, or exercises to maintain mobility may be all that is necessary. For more severe pain, a cortisone injection into the joint may provide relief, but this is usually only of temporary benefit. For pain and stiffness that is more severe and interferes with hand function, surgery may be required. Depending on which finger is affected, the surgery may be to fuse the joint (arthrodesis) or have surgery to do an artificial joint replacement (athroplasty).

☞ MALLET FINGER:

As described in the "Stiffness and Loss of Motion" section, a mallet finger deformity is a bend or droop of the end joint (distal interphalangeal joint) of a finger. It is caused by a rupture of the tendon that straightens the fingertip (extensor tendon) or a small bone fracture where the tendon is attached. Treatment is as described on page 37.

☞ BOUTONNIERE DEFORMITY:

Also as described in the "Stiffness and Loss of Motion" section, Boutonniere deformity is a bend in the middle finger joint (proximal interphalangeal joint) and results in an inability to straighten the joint because of a tendon rupture. Treatment for this condition is as described on page 38.

☞ SWAN-NECK DEFORMITY:

A Swan-Neck Deformity is a backward bend in the middle joint (proximal interphalangeal joint) of a finger due to an imbalance of tendon forces across the joint. This condition is frequently seen with rheumatoid or other forms of chronic arthritis. It may also develop over time as a result of an untreated mallet finger. The treatment of a swan-neck deformity is usually surgical and involves a somewhat complex transfer of portions of the extensor tendon, at times with tightening of the palm side of the middle finger joint capsule. This procedure is best done by a surgeon with specialized training in hand surgery.

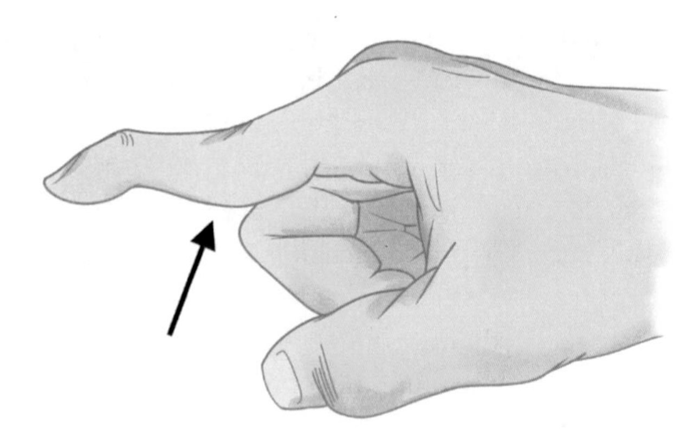

SWAN NECK DEFORMITY

In addition to hand deformities caused by arthritis, tendon injury, or bone fractures there is a host of hand deformities that are a result of various birth defects. These conditions are not particularly common, but they are especially important because they affect children, are of cosmetic concern, and in many cases, profoundly affect hand function. Deformities of this nature may show great variation, but the more common types include:

☞ CLINODACTYLY:

This is an angular bend in the little finger towards the thumb side of the hand. It usually occurs as an isolated deformity but can be part of a genetic disorder (Down's syndrome). It is painless and often minimal enough of a deformity to be barely recognized. Usually, the degree of angulation does not get better or worse over time. If the finger is at an angulation of less than 30 degrees, it will not interfere with function and requires no treatment. If the angulation is quite severe, interferes with function, and is of cosmetic concern, surgery may be advised. Surgery usually involves cutting the bone at the site of angulation and either removing a small wedge of the finger bone (middle phalanx) or opening a small wedge with a bone graft to straighten it. Once corrected, the deformity will not recur. Attempts to force the finger straight with a brace or splint will not be successful and should be avoided.

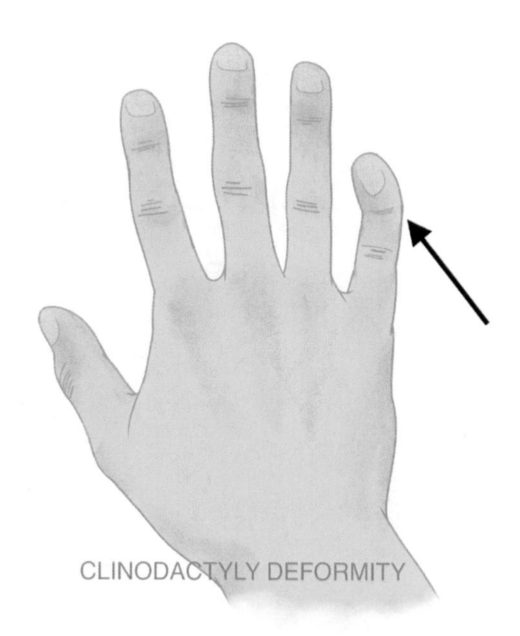

☞ CAMPTODACTYLY :

This is a birth defect marked by a bend (flexion) deformity of the finger middle joint. The deformity itself may seem similar to other flexion deformities of the middle joint (Boutonniere, Bouchard's node) discussed previously, but it is distinct in that it occurs in children without any tendon or joint injury. It is most common in the little finger, but it can affect other fingers or multiple fingers. It may not be obvious at birth, but does tend to progress with growth. It may occur without a family inheritance but can be a result of a broader genetic disorder. It is due to an imbalance of tendon forces across the middle finger joint with tendon forces that bend the middle joint being abnormally stronger than the tendons that straighten the joint.

Treatment of this condition depends on the degree of deformity and whether or not it is increasing rapidly. If the condition is mild and not worsening with growth, splinting the finger in a straight position may help to minimize the deformity. More often, though, this is not the case, and surgery to rebalance the tendon forces across the joint by a tendon transfer is the most effective treatment. If there is clear evidence that the deformity is worsening, surgical correction should not be delayed.

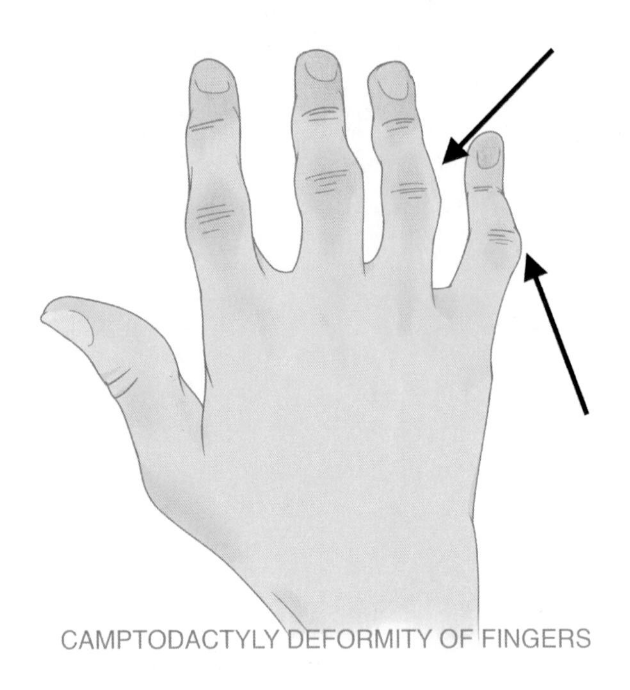

CAMPTODACTYLY DEFORMITY OF FINGERS

☞ SYNDACTYLY:

This is a birth defect where two or more fingers are webbed together. The web may extend the length of the involved fingers or only a short distance. The webbed tissue may be skin only (simple syndactyly) or may include shared nerves, blood vessels, tendons, and bones (complex syndactyly). This deformity can occur spontaneously or be family trait, or part of a syndrome with other abnormalities.

The treatment requires surgery to separate the joined fingers, and should be done by a medical professional with specialized training in hand surgery. The timing of surgery is best determined by whether the webbed connection is disturbing growth of the involved fingers. If so, surgery should be done in early childhood. However, the earlier that separation is done the more likely there will be some degree of recurrence of the webbing. Therefore, when finger growth is not being impaired a delay of surgery to later in childhood may be advised. It should also be noted that not all complex syndactyly cases can be safely separated depending on the extent that bones are joined together.

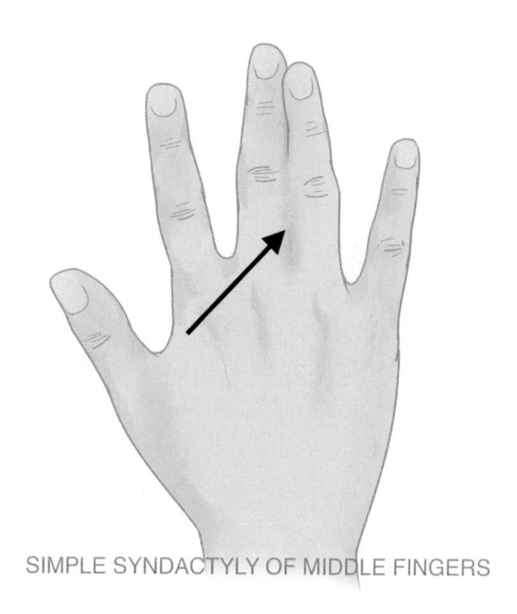

SIMPLE SYNDACTYLY OF MIDDLE FINGERS

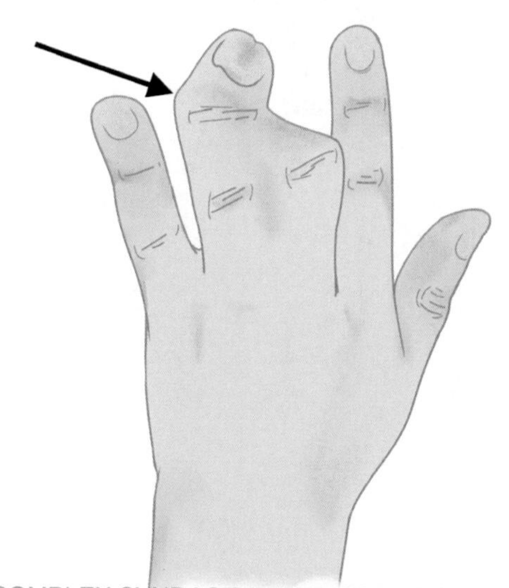

COMPLEX SYNDACTYLY OF MIDDLE FINGERS

☞ POLYDACTYLY:

Those with this deformity are born with more than four fingers and one thumb. The extra digits may be a well-developed normal-appearing finger, or what looks like a double thumb, two fingers joined together, or a small nubbin of skin and bone that doesn't resemble a finger at all. When the extra digit is on the little-finger side of the hand (ulnar), it is very often inherited with past generations or other family members sharing the deformity. When the extra digit is on the thumb side (radial), the condition is more often an isolated one without a family trait playing a role.

The treatment of polydactyly most often includes removal of the extra finger, especially if it is underdeveloped or just a nubbin. When the extra finger is normal in appearance and function, surgical removal is not an absolute necessity but usually is preferred for cosmetic reasons. When the extra digit is part of a syndactyly, the less-developed or partial digit will be separated and removed.

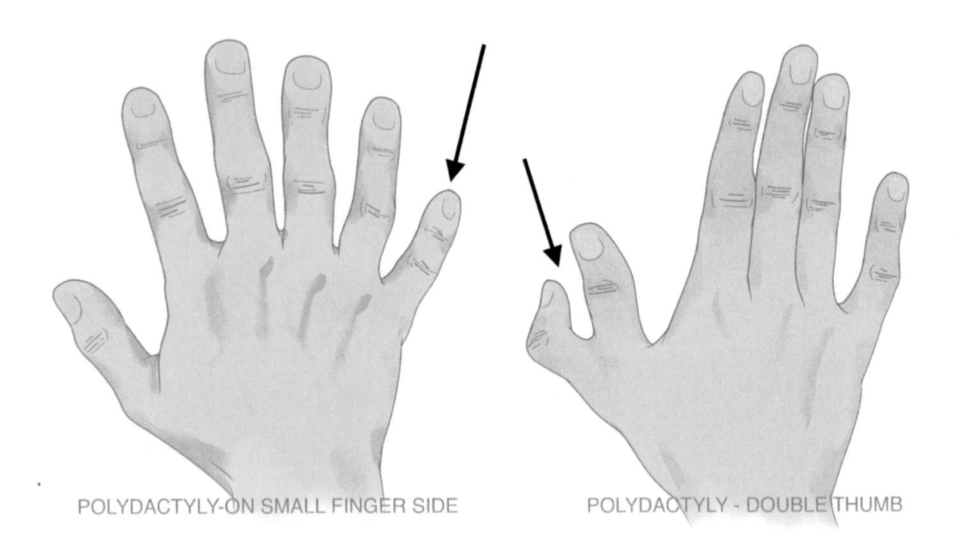

POLYDACTYLY-ON SMALL FINGER SIDE

POLYDACTYLY - DOUBLE THUMB

☞ BRACHYDACTYLY:

This deformity implies shortened fingers and/or thumbs. Brachydactyly may be an inherited deformity, and very often the shortened fingers are fully functional. However, some cases of brachydactyly are accompanied by other deformities like syndactyly or underdevelopment of the finger joints and tendons, resulting in both short and stiff fingers (symphalangism).

Treatment of brachydactyly is not always necessary if there is sufficient length and motion to permit grasp and pinch. When this is not the case and when there is a reasonable degree of mobility of the fingers, lengthening the shortened fingers using a special device (distraction lengthening) is often advised. When the shortened digit, and especially the thumb, is severely underdeveloped, reconstruction by transplanting one or more toes to the hand using microsurgery may be advised (toe-to-hand transfer).

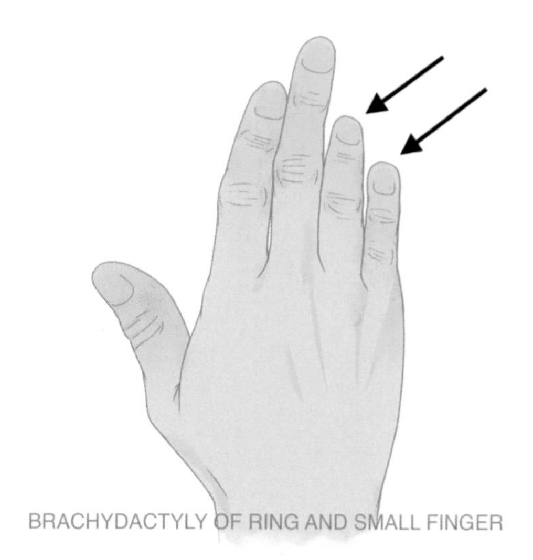

BRACHYDACTYLY OF RING AND SMALL FINGER

☞ CONSTRICTION RING SYNDROME:

This condition may appear as a wide variety of birth-related deformities. In its mildest form, it appears as a narrow depression around the circumference of the arm, wrist, hand, or finger as if a string had been tied tightly around the affected part. In more severe cases, the depression is deeper and with swelling (edema) of the limb or finger beyond the constriction. In the most severe cases, the constricting band may actually amputate the finger, hand, or arm before birth, and the infant will be born with missing fingers, hands, or forearms (or toes and legs). The cause of constricting ring syndrome is not known, but it is not considered hereditary.

Treatment for ring constriction is surgery. When there is complete amputation, the treatment needs to be individualized and may include the use of an artificial prosthesis or finger replacement through microsurgical toe transplantation (toe-to-hand transfer).

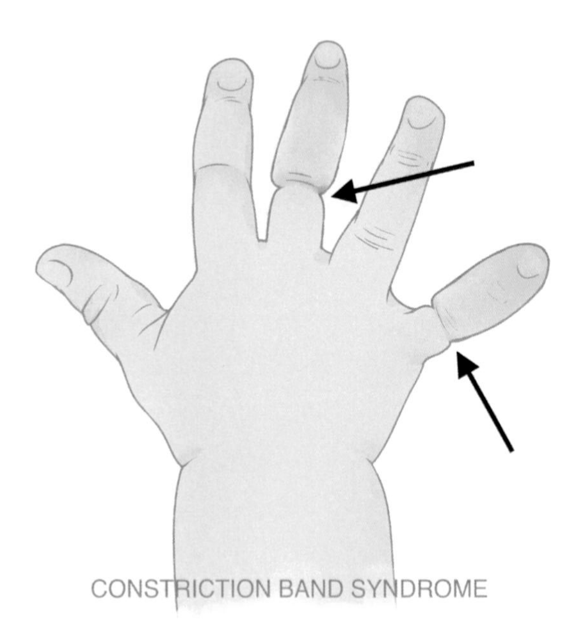

CONSTRICTION BAND SYNDROME

☞ RADIAL CLUB HAND:

This deformity is characterized by the underdevelopment of the thumb side of the hand, wrist, and forearm. It varies in severity with the mildest cases being a shortened, underdeveloped thumb. More typically, the thumb is underdeveloped or absent, the wrist is angulated, and the radius forearm bone is short. Radial Club Hand may be inherited or due to exposure to toxic agents or certain drugs (thalidomide) during early pregnancy. It may also be a component of certain syndromes that include heart, kidney, and blood disorders (Fanconi anemia). It affects both hands about half the time. Provided the elbow has adequate motion, the initial treatment is bracing to try to stretch the wrist into a more normal position. This is then followed by surgery to position the wrist straight in line with the forearm and to reconstruct a more normal, functioning thumb. When the thumb is very underdeveloped, it is usually removed and replaced using the index finger or by a toe-to-hand transfer.

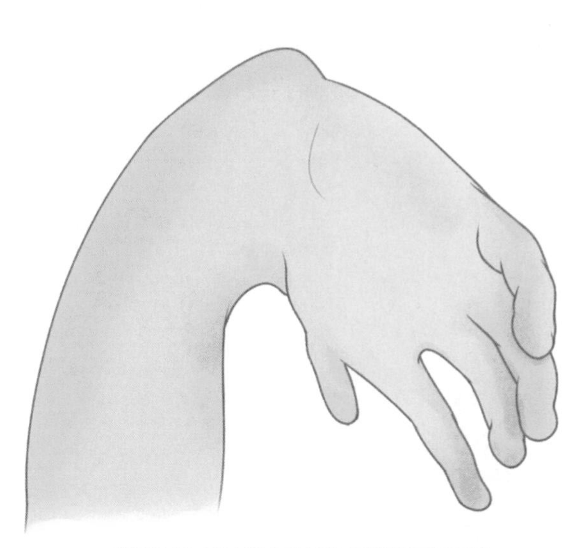

RADIAL CLUB HAND DEFORMITY

☞ MADELUNG'S DEFORMITY:

This deformity is restricted to the wrist, maintaining an otherwise normal hand. It is a disturbance of the growth plate (physis) of the forearm bone on the thumb side (radius). With this condition, the radius grows in an exaggerated palmar direction while the other forearm bone (ulna) grows in a normal manner. As a result, the hand appears to be shifted towards the palm and on the little finger side of the wrist, the end of the ulna appears as a distinct bony prominence. Madelung's deformity is not present at birth but becomes more obvious with growth in later adolescence and young adulthood. Its cause is unknown but it may be part of a genetic disorder and is more common in girls. In addition to the deformity, this condition can be a cause of wrist pain and weakness.

If the deformity is mild and not painful, treatment may be unnecessary. However, if more severe, surgery is the only effective treatment. This usually involves cutting the radius bone (osteotomy) near the wrist and repositioning it using a bone graft. In a younger child, surgery on the growth plate (physis) may be an option to avoid later osteotomy.

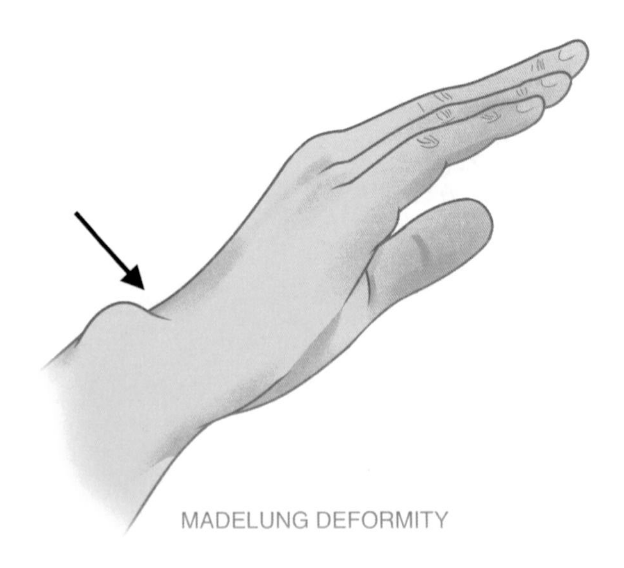

MADELUNG DEFORMITY

About the Author

The author, Michael B. Wood, MD graduated from the Faculty of Medicine of McGill University and completed training as an Orthopedic Surgeon at the Mayo Clinic, followed by additional training in Hand Surgery at the University of Louisville. His career as an Orthopedic Surgeon specializing in Hand Surgery and Reconstructive Microsurgery has been at the Mayo Clinic, Rochester, Minnesota (now retired). Dr. Wood is certified by the American Board of Orthopedic Surgery and also certified for additional qualifications for Surgery of the Hand. He is a member of the American Society for Surgery of the Hand and is past President of the American Society for Reconstructive Microsurgery. He has been recognized as a Pioneer of Hand Surgery by the International Federation for Surgery of the Hand. He currently is a Supplemental Consultant for Orthopedic Surgery at Mayo Clinic Florida and is Professor of Orthopedic Surgery at the Mayo Clinic Alix School of Medicine.